The New Detox Diet

The Complete Guide for Lifelong Vitality with Recipes, Menus, and Detox Plans

by Elson M. Haas, M.D., The Detox Doc®
with Daniella Chace, M.S., C.N.

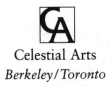

Celestial Arts
Berkeley/Toronto

Note: Ending our addictions is a serious undertaking. Going "cold turkey" from sedatives, stimulants, narcotics, and alcohol can have very serious consequences, including
seizures. There are many excellent doctors and facilities, including hospital detox centers, available to help us deal with drug and alcohol problems. This book is intended
to supplement, not substitute, the interventions of an experienced, professional health-
care practitioner. However, most of our habits are mild problems that can typically be
handled with will power and the guidance provided in this book.

Copyright © 2004 by Elson M. Haas, M.D.

Celestial Arts
P.O. Box 7123
Berkeley, California 94707
www.tenspeed.com

Distributed in Australia by Simon & Schuster Australia, in Canada by Ten Speed Press Canada, in New
Zealand by Southern Publishers Group, in South Africa by Real Books, and in the United Kingdom and
Europe by Airlift Book Company.

Cover design by Toni Tajima
Text design by Jeff Brandenburg, based on original design by Shelley Firth

Library of Congress Cataloging-in-Publication Data on file with the publisher.
1-58761-184-8

Printed in the United States
First printing this edition 2004.

1 2 3 4 5 6 7 8 9 10 — 09 08 07 06 05 04

Contents

Acknowledgments

◆

I first wish to thank all you readers for your support of my original *Detox Diet* book, for being aware of the importance of detoxification, and for spreading the word about this needed healing therapy. And thank you for acknowledging *The New Detox Diet* with your support.

Thank you **Bethany Argisle** for your continued contribution to my writing career and for keeping your awareness on the pulse of the Earth. And thank you for your writing touch and your many ideas for this new book.

A very special thank you to **Daniella Chace** for your spark and motivation for this book, and for your writing contribution, recipes, and smooth communications. Your research for the Resource Roundup will help our readers. And your writing additions to Chapters 4, 5, 12, and 13 are especially appreciated.

Thanks also to **Celestial Arts** for your support of *The New Detox Diet*—to **Jo Ann Deck**, our publisher, for your energetic encouragement; **Carrie Rodrigues**, our editor, for your professional guidance; and to **Toni Tajima**, for your cover design.

To Drs. **Franz Morrell** and **Alexander Wood** for the nutritional concepts that helped formulate the original Detox Diet.

Daniella Chace also had many associates who supported her contributions.

First, we thank **Richard Calcagno**, a patient of both of ours, for your request for a more extensive book about the detox process and the Detox Diet.

To **Lynn McCarthy**, friend and traveling companion, owner and great chef of Cottonwood Catering and Cooking School in Ketchum, ID for your culinary advice and recipe help.

To **Linda Landkammer**, for your research into the current studies regarding food combining, pH balancing, and live foods.

To Eden Foods, Seventh Generation, Mountain Green, and others for supplying us with non-toxic soap and information for this book.

Live clean and live healthy.

Renewal

◆

So many problems in western society come from excessive use of food and drugs. Abuses and addictions touch almost every person's life. I realize that these habits are as much a part of our social and cultural upbringing as they are our responses to dealing with the stresses of family, school, work, and society at large.

I don't want you to feel bad, weak, or inferior if any of these potentially destructive habits applies to you. I know the struggle between light and dark—between picking up that cup of coffee or glass of wine or that pack of cigarettes and the desire to stop. I also know that it is an incredible challenge to change anything—particularly to stop any addiction that we have relied upon for many years. I have seen that clearing our substance habits can be done—whether you or a loved one suffers—with greater attentiveness to our actions, with a gathering of our willpower, and with the support of our family and friends. I have also seen that it is very difficult without a willingness to deal openly with emotions and other adversaries that may block healing.

I do want to inspire and motivate you to change. The first principle for improving your health is to eliminate destructive habits. Even if you cannot believe that you can do without your substances completely, at least consider an "abuse break" and observe the change. Try a day or a week without caffeine, alcohol, or sugar, replacing them with a new habit—drinking water, walking, or swimming. Remember breathe deeply.

All addictions are ultimately self-destructive (some hurt others as well, such as alcohol and smoking). When you change that dynamic to self care—through both your internal healing process as well as with lifestyle and nutritional guidelines I describe in this book—you will begin to serve your body and life toward its higher potential. As you develop more nurturing and supportive habits—eating good food, exercising regularly, learning to cope with stress, and developing motivating attitudes—I know you will experience greater vitality, more positive relationships, and overall improved health.

Good luck on your journey.

Before You Begin

◆

As a physician, I am fascinated by the complexity, subtlety, and diversity of individual health habits—the combinations of various substances we imbibe and ingest. The spectrum of these substances includes the components of our diet (foods, drinks, chemicals), supplements (nutrients, herbs, and homeopathic remedies), drugs (prescription, over-the-counter, and recreational), and pollutants (herbicides, pesticides, hydrocarbons, and petrochemicals). These all are part of our possible choices and have effects on our life and health.

How do we develop our preferences? When do our preferences become needs? Why do our needs become addictions? Why do some of us become addicted while others can stop on our own? Our personality, upbringing, and environment influence our personal choice of substances. In exploring these concerns about abuse and the way it affects our health, I have developed a specific orientation and program for initial healing and detoxification. This process has evolved over my nearly thirty years as a naturally based, general health practitioner.

My overall understanding of symptoms and disease integrates both Western linear thinking and naturopathic approaches to health and illness. Problems with the body and mind often arise from either deficiency (when we are not acquiring sufficient nutrients to meet our bodily needs) and/or congestion (when our intake is excessive). Congestion involves both reduced elimination function and an over-consumption of food, or substances, such as caffeine, alcohol, nicotine, refined sugar, and chemicals from home cleaners to freeway fumes.

People who are deficient may experience problems such as fatigue, coldness, hair loss, or dry skin. They need to be nourished with wholesome foods (and supportive relationships) that aid healing. However, congestive problems are more common in Western, industrialized countries. Many of our acute and chronic diseases result from clogged tissues, suffocated cells, and subsequent loss of vital energy. Frequent colds and flus, cancer, cardiovascular diseases, arthritis, and allergies are all consequences of congestive disorders. These medical problems may be prevented or treated through a process of cleansing, fasting, and detoxification. These represent different degrees of a process that reduces toxin intake and enhances toxin elimination, making way for health and healing to occur.

All of the programs contained in this book combine aspects of these fasting and detoxification processes. I have written specific programs for dealing with Sugar, Nicotine, Alcohol, Caffeine, and Chemicals (drugs)—what I call SNACCs. In each program, I discuss the physiological actions and reactions involved, the hazards and ill effects of the substance, and the methods for handling and clearing these adverse habits.

The beginning of the process for healing our abuses requires motivation from within to change unwanted habits. This often requires us to address the underlying emotions that may perpetuate the problem. A good counselor or therapist or a compassionate supportive friend can be helpful to support this healing process. Overall, we must create a workable plan and gather our will power to begin. The Detox Diet and other purifying programs discussed throughout this book alkalize the body, help us feel better quickly, and lessen feelings of withdrawal. Water, exercise, and many nutritional and herbal supplements also support the detoxification process.

A few simple tenets of natural medical practice may help clarify for you this book's approach:

1. The primary cause of disease is the accumulation of unnecessary wastes that are not properly eliminated, resulting in poison retention and subsequent health problems.

2. Your body is designed to support optimal function. Listen to its signals.

3. Given the proper environment, your body has the power (and likelihood) to heal itself and return to its normal healthy state.

I believe that patients and physicians do best when oriented to live and practice with a commonsense approach that first looks at lifestyle as a place to promote rejuvenation, then to natural therapies, and finally to pharmaceutical drugs and surgery, which are appropriate when a situation is acute or severe or if natural therapies are not working. Lifestyle factors include diet, exercise, stress management, and attitudes. Natural therapies include supplements, herbs, homeopathics, and hands-on healing such as massage, osteopathy, and chiropractic care. Nutritional awareness and practice aid you in both preventing disease and health recovery.

Put simply, the key to maintaining metabolic balance is to maximize nutrition and to eliminate toxins.

My goal is to place your health and that of your family back into your own hands. In fact, so much of your health is up to you. Take the initiative to do what you can to be vital and healthy. It is really worth it!

Be clean and clear, healthy and free,

Dr. Elson M. Haas

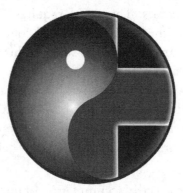

Preface

◆

When I did my first fast with the "Master Cleanser" in 1976, I would never have thought or believed that the idea of cleansing and detoxification would become so important in my life and career. Well, it makes perfect sense given the toxic times in which we live where we are exposed to chemicals in our basic elements of air, water, and food, with some extra food pollutants thrown in the mix. Nowadays, the topic of detoxification is a crucial one and most important to the health of many.

That is basically why my simple book *The Detox Diet* has been so popular. It is a crucial message and guide for inspiring people to awaken to a wiser, healthier lifestyle. *The Detox Diet* and its transformative guidelines have been an empowering tool in my medical practice for the past twenty years with literally thousands of patients experiencing benefits. This book, originally published in late 1996, has also been used by many other physicians and natural health practitioners for themselves and their patients or clients. In fact, that's the way I connected with nutritionist and author Daniella Chace and her work in Sun Valley, Idaho. She had followed and used my book with her clients and also guided detox groups with consistently wonderful results. In our initial discussions, she believed, as I did, that with our experiences we could make the original text, already simple to follow, even more thorough and user-friendly. My publisher, Celestial Arts in Berkeley, California, is typically open to updates, so they were very supportive.

And now you have in your hands this new, more extensive detox book, which includes additional options for detox, even clearer guidelines, and many clean and tasty recipes. Working with Daniella has been smooth and easy. Using modern technology, we were able to pass chapters and edits back and forth over the Internet, and then pass them onto Carrie Rodrigues, our editor at Celestial, saving postage, paper, and trees.

And my longtime book associate and "user friendly queen", Bethany Argisle, has included some personal stories about what it's like to be a smoker or coffee drinker and the challenge of letting these habits go. I hope this will inspire our readers to journal their personal experience for themselves, since *The New Detox Diet* process is quite a personal and individual one moment by moment, season after season. This book will motivate and guide you in the how-tos, and can be used on a regular basis.

So, give it a go. You have lots more tips on how to detox, more choices in your diet options for cleansing your body and life, and many recipes to make this crucial health transformation process easier to follow and even tastier to eat.

The New Detox Diet experience is an important step toward being your own best doctor.

Elson Haas, M.D., The Detox Doc®
June, 2004
www.elsonhaas.com

Note: This book is a new and expanded version of *The Detox Diet*. Daniella Chace has helped in the expansion. She has contributed original writings, particularly in Chapters 4, 5, 12, and 13. However, the text, where the pronoun "I" is used refers to writing and suggestions from Dr. Elson Haas. Use this book toward your good health.

Introduction to Detox

◆

by Daniella Chace, M.S., C.N.

In the years that I spent on campus at Bastyr University, while earning my Bachelor's and Master's degrees, I did my classroom and clinical work alongside naturopathic, Oriental medicine, and Ayurvedic students. This is where I learned the value of taking a holistic approach to health and nutrition. To treat an individual holistically means to take into consideration all aspects of that individual including mind and body, seeing to both their emotional and nutritional needs. When you look at health issues this way, one of the first steps is to remove all of the things that hinder health, and this includes attitudes as well as all the substances or chemicals we consume that create toxicity.

Over the last decade in my nutrition consultation practice I have learned that when my clients are willing to detox from substances and chemically laden foods, they experience quicker and much more substantial results. Being steeped in the knowledge that most health problems stem from a life imbalance (such as too much junk and too little nutrient-rich foods), I was thrilled to connect with Dr. Elson Haas, whose clinical work with detoxification serves as examples for students at Bastyr University. We used his valuable book *Staying Healthy with Nutrition* as our course textbook.

Dr. Haas and I both lead detox groups in our hometowns of San Rafael, California, and Sun Valley, Idaho, respectively. Together we bring to this newly revised book many lessons we learned from our clients and class participants. From this experience, I saw a need for a wider range of Detox Diets to meet individual goals. For example, many people are athletic, especially in the high mountain valley where I live, and have a higher caloric need throughout their cleansing programs.

The most common request that came from my classes has been for more guidance after our cleansing program. Those who go through detoxification generally feel so good that they want to know how they can continue to feel that way when they go back to their daily diet. Well, that's why our health plan encourages positive habit changes and better food choices, which takes conscientious shopping and healthier preparation. To address this need, Elson and I developed a nutrient-dense diet that helps people stay in that "post-detox purity" while providing enough calories for everyday life.

The most exciting observation for me has been to see how much more quickly we all heal when we detox as part of our treatment program. This applies to almost all illnesses. Many people have either had the attitude that they needed to put up with toxicity symptoms, such as headaches, joint pain, fatigue, digestive problems, and so on, or they have used medications as a band-aid to mask the symptoms of toxicity. They, unfortunately, have resolved themselves to being "unwell" as if it was an unavoidable part of aging.

It's so satisfying to hear how my clients' lives change after they complete a "cleanse." They usually report that it feels too good to be true and that it has taken them a few weeks to get used to the feeling of having a high energy level again. The analogy I hear most often is that when your body is not dealing with toxins, you feel like a kid again, when we last knew what being toxin-free felt like.

I wish you all an exciting journey throughout your Detox Diet! When you find that clean, high energy person you never thought you would be again, take hold and make this a new way of living throughout your life!

In health,

Daniella Chace, nutritionist

www.daniellachace.com

CHAPTER ONE

Gastrointestinal Health

Gastrointestinal function and ecology are at the core of human health. In other words, how well we are able to digest and absorb our food, along with the levels of good and potentially harmful bacteria that live in our bowel, definitely influence our overall health and well-being. Likewise, the structure and functions of the intestines determine total body toxin load and are essential to the process of detoxification. Cleansing and healing the gastrointestinal (GI) tract (especially the colon) provide a base for effective detoxification. The liver has many functions as part of the GI tract. Even though it does so much more in terms of body function, not stressing our liver and supporting both its rest and detoxification processes are important as well.

"We are what we eat and assimilate, and not what we eliminate," is really saying that our GI tract function is vital to the process of nourishing our body and controlling toxicity through elimination, a process that only ends in the colon. Furthermore,

SOME IMPRESSIVE GI TRACT FACTS

- The total GI mucosal surface is made up of many microscopic crypts and crevices, most of which are in the small intestine and have the interactive area equivalent to the size of a tennis court.

- There are more bacteria (10^{12}) in a gram of stool than there are stars in the known universe.

- The microbes of the GI tract constitute a very metabolically active area of the body, second only to the liver.

- The total weight of the bacteria located in the colon of the average human equals approximately five pounds (or about the weight of our liver).

- The digestive organs manufacture nearly a gallon of juices per day to help digest and utilize the food we eat.

we must regularly cleanse the intestinal system to effectively detoxify the body. Specific therapies are discussed throughout this book; in this chapter, there is a basic discussion of the GI tract process and its contribution to overall health—a relationship often overlooked in Western medicine.

In this model (which I call Functional Integrated Medicine), the function, ecology, and permeability of the GI tract are crucial to the health of each patient. *Dysbiosis* is the term used to describe an imbalance of GI function (specifically, incomplete food digestion and assimilation), and especially, its microbial populations. Functional Integrated Medicine works with the theory that imbalance in a body system precedes abnormal function; abnormal function precedes symptoms; and symptoms, left unchecked, can precede pathology. This is why the GI tract is assessed for dysbiosis, and particularly an imbalance in the gut bacteria.

Therefore, in order to prevent pathology, normal functioning must be restored. This is particularly true of the GI tract. When this concept of prevention is incorporated into mainstream medicine, we will keep people healthier longer and prevent disease by evaluating and maintaining proper internal function and environment. Fortunately, this shift in lifestyle approach is gaining momentum around the country.

The GI tract is composed of the mouth and teeth, the esophagus and stomach, and the small intestine (duodenum, jejunum, and ileum) and large intestine (colon). Its proper function begins with **adequate chewing,** which is essential for good nutrition and health. Other digestive organs include the salivary glands, pancreas, gall bladder, GI mucous glands, and liver. Salivary enzymes begin digestion and the process is continued by hydrochloric acid in the stomach, plus the many pancreatic enzymes that are released into the upper small intestine. Finally, the gall bladder releases bile to promote fat digestion. Assimilation of most nutrients occurs in the small intestine; the colon absorbs water, bile salts, and a few other substances in order to prepare the remainder of the colonic contents for elimination.

Regular elimination is also crucial to overall health and control of the level of toxicity in the body—constipation is actually a greater problem than most doctors and patients realize. Hydration, diet, level of physical activity, and stress all affect our eliminative function.

Health and proper functional integrity of the huge mucosal membrane surface area of the GI tract allows the proper assimilation of nutrients. Even minor disruptions related to inflammation or infection may cause abnormal absorption and increased barrier permeability. With increased intestinal permeability, absorption goes out of balance and larger-than-normal molecules get absorbed, which can cause allergic reactions and other abnormal immune responses. There is a delicate balance between the assimilation of needed nutrients and the exclusion of toxic substances. Abnormal organisms within the intestinal lumen may also produce toxins that can significantly affect mental and physical health. Also, certain pathogens within the GI tract may generate autoimmune reactions in the particularly vulnerable environment of the small bowel, where the majority of our immune cells are located.

Problems of dysbiosis, abnormal GI mucosal permeability, infection, and inflammation are exceedingly common and may cause both gastrointestinal complaints and other health concerns.

The GI tract is stressed and otherwise adversely affected by the following:

- refined foods and sugar
- excess fatty and rich foods
- overeating and failing to chew more than once or twice per mouthful of food
- drinking too much with meals, thus diluting our digestive juices and reducing our ability to properly break down food
- food chemicals, pesticides, and environmental toxins
- the persistent use of alcohol, caffeine, and nicotine
- use of prescription, over-the-counter, and recreational drugs
- lack of fiber and whole foods, specifically lacking fresh fruits, vegetables, whole grains, and legumes in the diet
- eating too many different kinds of foods at a time and doing so over the course of many years (one of the key causes of obesity and a chronic breakdown of digestive health and function)

The GI tract is especially sensitive to emotional turmoil. A stressful lifestyle may adversely affect motility, digestive enzyme output, and overall function. Over 30 gut hormones have been identified, many of which also act as neurotransmitters. Chemical exposure (specifically ingested chemicals), travel, eating out often, and subsequent parasitic infections, or the overuse of antibiotics can cause intestinal dysfunction and disease. It may take years for the gut to recover from this kind of damage.

It is also important to maintain proper levels of friendly bacteria within the colon and make sure that their numbers decrease in concentration when progressing up the GI tract into the small intestine or stomach. Overgrowth of abnormal bacteria, fermenting yeasts, and parasites can disturb GI function causing inflammation along the sensitive mucous membrane of the GI tract and thereby adversely affecting the assimilation of food and nutrients.

Abnormal permeability, often called "leaky gut," creates GI imbalance, which can lead to systemic disease. Overconsumption of non-nutrient compounds and underconsumption or under assimilation of required nutrients may produce deficiencies and may lead to allergies or other immune system problems. Inflammation or infection in the GI tract, food allergies, and the overuse of alcohol and non-steroid anti-inflammatory drugs (NSAIDs) can all cause problems with permeability. Disorders such as irritable bowel syndrome (IBS), Crohn's disease, rheumatoid arthritis, and HIV infections are frequently associated with leaky gut and permeability problems. A common condition involves fermentation from yeast overgrowth, specifically *Candida albicans* and other related Candida species, which can lead to a large variety of symptoms and which are often associated with permeability problems.

There are literally billions of microorganisms inhabiting the healthy GI tract. Friendly ones include *E. coli* (the bacteria *Escherichia coli*), various streptococci, and *Lactobacillus acidophilus,* as well as *Lactobacillus bifidis* (bifidobacteria), which is predominant in infants and children. However, many other undesirable organisms reside in the GI tract, particularly in the large intestine. These can include yeasts, abnormal bacteria such as *Klebsiella* (not always pathogenic) and *Citrobacter* species, a variety of pathogenic parasites that include *Giardia lamblia* and *Blastocystis hominis,* and amoebas such as histolytica, hartmani, and coli.

HEALING THE GI TRACT

An effective way to think about and heal the gastrointestinal tract has been developed and taught by Jeff Bland, Ph.D., Leo Galland, M.D., and others in their nutritional education seminars. This is an aspect of Functional or Physiological Medicine. Preventive Medicine focuses on basic functions within the body, balancing or rebalancing them when they are not right through the use of supportive nutrients and appropriate natural substances. This is similar to OrthoMolecular Medicine, a concept coined by Linus Pauling with whom Dr. Bland worked for a number of years. Currently, Dr. Bland and his team at Metagenics (previously HealthComm) in Gig Harbor, Washington, are working to find better ways to assess, heal, and support GI anatomy and physiology as a way to remedy illness and generate health.

There have been a number of new tests developed in the last decade or two that look at digestion and assimilation, GI mucosal surface health, and the presence or absence of appropriate or pathogenic bacteria, yeasts, and parasites. Several licensed laboratories across the country (particularly Great Smokies (Genova) Diagnostic Lab in Asheville, North Carolina) have led the way in developing very useful, clinically significant tests that follow along with the basic medical GI tests.

GASTROINTESTINAL TESTS

Allopathic Medical Tests

1. Upper GI, or the Barium Swallow, X-Ray Study

A series of x-rays are taken (viewed with dye) from the mouth to the small intestine. This is useful for identifying anatomical and motility problems as significant problems like gastric or peptic ulcers, hiatal hernias, and tumors within (or pushing into) the upper GI tract are detected. Concerns with this test and the barium enema include the x-ray exposure, constipation from the relatively nontoxic dye (which only rarely causes reactions), and fluid/nutrient imbalance resulting from the enemas and oral purgatives used in preparation for these tests. Cleansing the bowels after the tests by drinking water and taking vitamin C will help counter some of the radiation and toxin exposure.

2. The Barium Enema

This rather unpleasant test involves the slow injection of a highly pressurized enema into a cleaned-out colon to examine the area from rectum to small intestine. It is used to diagnose ulcerative colitis in progressed stages, tumors (both benign and cancerous), and misshapen colons, which are often the result of many years of poor diet and constipation.

3. Scopes: Gastroscopy, Colonoscopy, and Sigmoidoscopy

The gastroscope is a fiberoptic tube that is inserted through the mouth to view the esophagus, stomach, and pyloric area. The colonoscope is inserted through the anus and travels around the colon. Both scopes are used to search out inflammation, polyps, tumors, or ulcers. A less comprehensive test employs a flexible sigmoidoscope, which does not travel as far around the colon yet is a simpler office procedure than the colonoscopy, which usually is done in outpatient surgery under moderate anesthesia. (The "silver tube" or sigmoidoscope is a rigid instrument used to assess the rectum and sigmoid colon only. This test was more painful and less helpful and has been replaced by the flexible tube.) The obvious advantage of the scopes for testing is the total avoidance of any exposure to radiation. Biopsies or even complete excisions can be performed utilizing the instruments, often avoiding, or at least postponing, more invasive surgery. These procedures can, however, be quite painful, and doctors often give multiple anti-pain and tranquilizing drugs, or even general anesthesia, from which it may take several days for some people to recover.

Functional GI Tests

4. CDSA—Comprehensive Digestive Stool Analysis (including the new CDSA 2.0 from Great Smokies Diagnostic Labs.)

This simple assessment has been a medical breakthrough. A stool is collected and mailed overnight to a lab where it is evaluated for digestion of protein, vegetable matter and starch, and fatty acids. Cutting-edge markers for intestinal immune function such as *calprotectin* and *eosinophil protein* X are included in the test. Exocrine pancreatic function (that part associated with digestion) is measured by an analyte called *pancreatic elastase 1*. In addition, a number of markers that not only address proper digestive function but also give the doctor insight into the patient's risk for colon cancer (the second leading cause of cancer in our country) are integral to the test. These include stool pH, beta-glucuronidase, butyrate, and short-chain fatty acids. Culturing the stool is done to identify both normal and abnormal bacteria and yeast or fungus. The stool is also tested for the presence or absence of parasites. If any abnormal organisms are detected, sensitivity testing is done with both natural substances (such as garlic, plant tannins, grapefruit seed extract, oregano oil, and caprylic acid) and pharmaceutical agents (such as antibiotics and antifungals) to determine which agents kill or inhibit the growth of the detected organism. This allows the practitioner and patient to select the right treatment for the particular condition. This information provides us with a therapeutic plan that involves the *removal* of abnormal organisms, *replacement* of diminished enzymes or hydrochloric acid, *reinoculation* with appropriate helpful microorganisms (probiotics), and *repair* of the GI mucosa. This constitutes the 4R program, which is discussed later in this chapter as "the 5R program," with the addition of *rebalancing* diet and lifestyle. There are no side effects or medical concerns with the

CDSA or the Parasite Study other than the psychological discomfort that some people experience from having to handle their own feces. This test may also involve a purged sample in which we drink something like magnesium citrate or phospho-soda to cause loose bowels since some parasites can live higher up in the intestines and a standard stool sample might not provide enough organisms to identify them. This part of the test can be uncomfortable and cause loose bowels temporarily.

5. Parasite Study

Certain laboratories specialize in identifying parasitic infections through stool exams. These exams require a loose or a special "purged" stool collection—a watery sample that is observed under a special microscope. (The purging process may cause some diarrhea, but its mildly cleansing effect may have some benefit as well.) These parasitic infections are quite common, even in people who do not travel outside the United States. The labs I currently use are the Institute for Parasitic Diseases (IPD) in Phoenix, Arizona, and Great Smokies Diagnostic Labs in Asheville, North Carolina. Their findings often correlate well with clinical symptoms. I look for parasites in anyone who presents with GI dysfunction (especially pain, gas, bloating, and nausea), allergies, fatigue, insomnia, teeth grinding at night, anxiety, or other psycho-emotional symptoms.

6. Intestinal Permeability

This is a simple test that measures the small intestine's ability to absorb needed nutrients and discriminate against harmful substances. After the patient drinks a solution composed of two sugars (lactulose and mannitol), a urine sample is collected and the levels of these two sugars are measured. Mannitol is normally absorbed at approximately 20 percent, while lactulose should be absorbed very little, if at all. People with increased intestinal permeability absorb excess lactulose. This suggests that they also inappropriately absorb other larger molecules due to damaged intestinal walls. Such absorption can cause secondary immunologic reactions and subsequent food allergies and intolerance. Working the 5R program will often normalize intestinal permeability. This test and the Breath Test have no side effects at all. The two mostly non-absorbable sugars mentioned above occasionally cause temporarily loose bowels.

7. Breath Test for Small Intestine Bacterial Overgrowth

This test measures levels of hydrogen and methane gases in breath samples to assess bacterial overgrowth in the small intestine. Although this problem is more common in the elderly, it should be considered for anyone with gas, bloating, diarrhea, chronic halitosis (bad breath), or carbohydrate intolerance. Bacterial overgrowth can compromise health both in the GI tract and throughout the body and can lead to malabsorption, failure to thrive, anemia, weakened immunity, and increased risk of colon cancer (intestinal bacteria may produce additional carcinogens). This test is suggested when the standard 5R approach is not working effectively enough.

8. Detoxification Profile

This is a relatively new procedure that tests the detoxification functions of the liver. The body must be able to metabolize and clear xenobiotics (environmental chemicals), endotoxins (generated from gut flora), and our own waste products of metabolism (including hormones and cholesterol). The Detoxification Profile measures two primary liver pathways: Phase I, oxidation and reduction, such as in caffeine metabolism, and Phase II, glycine, glutathione, and sulfate conjugation, as well as glucuronidation. Each demonstrates the patient's ability or inability to detoxify certain types of chemicals. Standardized test doses of caffeine, aspirin, and acetaminophen are given, and then both salivary and urine samples are taken and studied to identify the level of detoxification. The only concern with this test would be any adverse reactions to the testing agents, which are taken and studied to identify the level of detoxification.

I use these tests judiciously whenever I see a patient with gastrointestinal concerns or systemic symptoms correlated with gastrointestinal dysbiosis, inflammation, or toxicity. After gathering information from these tests, I decide upon a course of therapy, which is often multidisciplinary in its approach. Detoxification practices—the focus of this book—are an important first step in healing, since many diseases are related to congestion and toxicity from excessive or persistent intake and improper elimination.

A therapeutic regimen often includes dietary changes such as avoiding certain foods or food groups and adding more fresh, high-fiber and low-fat fruits, vegetables, and whole grains. I also address abusive habits and try to motivate my patients to give this therapy approach a fair chance. Most modern-day abuses—Sugar, Nicotine, Alcohol, Caffeine, and Chemicals—are psychoactive substances that have mental and emotional effects. I believe that giving up at least the habitual use of these SNACCs (as I call them) is extremely important. I also promote chewing your food thoroughly along with regular and systematic undereating. **If we make what we eat wholesome and nourishing, we will not only add years to our lives, but life to our years.** Choosing the right foods and diet for ourselves, our activity level, and the climate in which we live are key guidelines for a healthy GI tract.

Other Lifestyle and Therapeutic Activities for GI Health

1. Learn to manage stress. Our sensitive digestive tract works better when we are calm, so don't hold onto and chew emotions.

2. Set up and do a regular exercise program. Exercise improves digestive functions, stimulates lymphatic flow, and supports immune function.

3. Utilize and experience musculoskeletal therapies. This may involve osteopathic or chiropractic realignment of the spine and massage treatments.

4. Use nutritional supplements and herbs. (See the following list for those supplements that support the GI tract health.)

5. Seek professional advice on the use of pharmaceutical (or herbal) agents to remove infectious and harmful organisms, including abnormal bacteria, yeasts, and parasites.

THE 5R PLAN

The 5R Gastrointestinal Support Plan is a progressive therapeutic program normalizes the function, environment, and tissue health of the GI tract and must be tailored to the individual according to his or her particular evaluation.

The 5R steps are the following:

1. Rebalance—your diet, your lifestyle, and your life. (This "R" was added to Dr. Bland's 4R Plan by my associate, Scott V. Anderson, M.D.) This is important as these areas contribute to health and the state of the digestive tract. Staying away from sugar, refined foods, and irritating substances such as caffeine and alcohol can make a big difference. Learning to deal with stress and developing coping and relaxation skills can help rebalance the GI tract biochemistry and support better digestion and assimilation.

Changing habits is not easy. A nutritional counselor, psychologist, or hypnotherapist can help by making us aware of the way old conditioning undermines our new positive health habits.

2. Remove—any offending organisms, particularly pathogenic microbes and/or any food antigens that cause allergic and immunologic reactions.

At this therapeutic level, we evaluate and treat any organisms that do not belong in the human GI tract. These include *Giardia lamblia,* abnormal types or levels of yeast organisms such as *Candida albicans,* and bacterial pathogens. Sensitivity testing (finding what therapeutic agents eliminate the specific microbe) can be done on most of these organisms to find the appropriate pharmaceutical or natural medications. Often, there is more than one type of pathogen, and a combination of medications may be needed. Treatments will vary according to the practitioner's training. One useful book is *Guess What Came to Dinner* by Ann Louise Gittleman; the author discusses the great prevalence of parasitic disease and the best ways, both natural and pharmaceutical, to treat each specific parasite. You can also see the Centers for Disease Control's website (www.CDC.gov) for the latest medical treatments on parasites.

We also encourage following an elimination diet that avoids allergenic, reactive foods and removes irritating substances such as caffeine, alcohol, refined sugar, and flour. Following a "hypoallergenic" diet involves eliminating common food allergens such as cow's milk, eggs, gluten grains (wheat, rye, barley, and oats), chocolate, coffee, and peanuts (and even soy products in some people). Any food that is consumed regularly or overconsumed should also be eliminated. A diet of fruits, vegetables, rice and beans, some nuts and seeds, fish, and poultry is usually an improvement for most people, producing a reduction of symptoms and an increase in energy.

3. Replace—inadequate amounts of hydrochloric acid (HCl), digestive enzymes, and pancreatic products. Fiber supplementation may also be necessary.

Nutritional substances in this category aid in food breakdown and in its subsequent absorption into the bloodstream for travel to the metabolic factory of the liver. Proper digestion reduces the allergenic and inflammatory effects that occur from larger, more complex molecules.

The CDSA (Comprehensive Digestive Stool Analysis, see page 18) helps identify digestion weaknesses and guides the practitioner and patient toward the proper replacement support. For instance, enzyme or hydrochloric acid insufficiency is common in people who experience indigestion, gas and bloating, belching and flatulence, and the presence of food particles in the stool. Yeast overgrowth is another problem and should be ruled out prior to treatment.

Replacement products are categorized as follows:
• Betaine and other forms of HCl
• Plant-derived digestive enzymes (proteases, amylases, lipases, and cellulases)
• Animal-derived enzymes (proteases, amylases, lipases, and elastases)
• Microbe-derived digestive enzymes
• Lactase enzyme supplements
• Fiber, both soluble and insoluble

4. Reinoculation—refers to the reintroduction or "reflorastation" of desirable bacterial flora as well as special nutrients such as fructooligosaccharides (FOS), which support the growth and function of friendly microorganisms.

Reinoculation includes supplementation of symbiotic bacteria normally present in the healthy GI tract. These bacteria, called "probiotics," include *Lactobacillus acidophilus* (also bulgaricus and thermophilus) and *Bifidobacteria bifidus* (also longum, infantis, and breve). They are predominant in the gut of young, healthy people but often decrease with age, especially with the use of antibiotics, exposure to toxic chemicals and metals, and substance abuse (particularly alcohol and caffeine). Also, recurrent infections (including GI pathogenic and parasitic infections), abnormal intestinal pH, lowered immune status, and abnormal digestion may contribute to imbalanced flora.

A second CDSA can determine whether or not this reflorastation has been successful. The supplements used should be viable strains of the microbes stated above and should be stored and shipped at cool temperatures. Probiotics are available primarily in powder form and as capsules or tablets, although cultured yogurt or milk products also contain some Lactobacilli species.

5. Repair—means providing nutritional support for the regeneration and healing of the gastrointestinal lining and is probably the most important component of the 5R Program.

The GI mucosal cells represent the largest mass of biochemically active and proliferating cells in the body. Repair is needed when the structure or function of the gastrointestinal mucosa loses its integrity. Both the CDSA and Permeability tests will help identify disrepair or dysbiosis. Loss of integrity can result from infection (particularly from parasites or yeast), food allergy, chronic nutritional deficiency, chemical exposure, inflammatory bowel disease, and general dysbiosis.

Proper detoxification begins with understanding gastrointestinal function and its effect on overall health. You will find that these guidelines, when combined with regular exercise, will improve your health, vitality, and the functioning of your gastrointestinal tract. This, in turn, reduces the chance of degenerative and chronic diseases, and helps slow the aging process. **Remember, prevention is the key!**

Some of the important nutrients for healing the GI tract include the amino acid L-glutamine, pantothenic acid, zinc, vitamin A, antioxidants (such as vitamins C and E, beta-carotene, and selenium), the bioflavonoid quercetin, essential fatty acids, inulin, and fiber (particularly the soluble kind). Herbs such as aloe vera, licorice root, and marshmallow root also have positive healing effects on the mucosal lining of the gastrointestinal tract. These nutrients play a key role in GI mucosal cell differentiation, growth, function, and repair. The following chart describes these important nutrients.

NUTRIENTS FOR HEALING THE GI TRACT

For further, in-depth discussions of these important nutrients, see *Staying Healthy with Nutrition.*

1. **L-glutamine** is a nonessential amino acid used as fuel by active cells, particularly the enterocytes (mucosal lining cells) of the GI tract. Extra L-glutamine is needed to heal the GI tract during disease.

2. **Pantothenic Acid (vitamin B5)** is necessary for protein synthesis and ATP energy production, both of which are involved in the tissue healing process. It is also works with vitamin C to handle stress and support the adrenals.

3. **Ascorbic Acid (vitamin C)** is essential for collagen formation, which is the basis for connective tissue repair, wound healing, and general tissue strength. It also works as an antioxidant to counter free radicals that can damage and inflame tissues.

4. **Vitamin A (retinol) and Beta-Carotene,** the nontoxic precursor of vitamin A, is needed for normal growth, function, and repair of epithelial cells, including those in the GI mucosa. Taking both nutrients ensures proper levels of vitamin A.

5. **Vitamin E** is an essential antioxidant that defends cell membrane integrity and function, thus helping to protect active enzyme systems within the cells.

6. **Zinc** (picolinate, as one bioavailable example) is essential to tissue health and repair, enzyme function, the integrity of the cell membrane structure, and cell replication. All of these processes are needed for the function and repair of the GI lining. Research from France indicates that zinc can be unusually effective in healing GI tissue inflammation.

7. **Selenium** is an important antioxidant for chemical detoxification, which protects GI tract cells from damage and allows appropriate repair.

8. **Quercetin** is a bioflavonoid with antihistamine and anti-inflammatory effects, useful in reducing food allergy reactions and helping in tissue repair.

---

9. **Essential Fatty Acids (EFAs)** help to maintain the integrity of cell membranes and protect and heal the cells and tissues. Good sources include Gamma Linolenic Acid (GLA) from evening primrose oil and borage oil, as well as Eicosapentaenoic Acid (EPA) and Docosahexaenoic Acid (DHA) from fish oils, and to a lesser degree from other cold pressed, unheated vegetable oils. Fresh organic flaxseed oil offers a good source of EFAs.

10. **Inulin** is a storage carbohydrate found in onions and Jerusalem artichokes that acts as fuel for colon epithelial cells and promotes healing and energy generation.

11. **Aloe Vera,** in its purified and extracted juice form, is both soothing and healing to the GI tract mucosa and tissue.

12. **Licorice Root and DGL (deglycirrhized licorice)** has an anti-inflammatory effect in the GI tract. DGL is particularly helpful in healing ulcers and other stomach inflammations.

13. **Marshmallow root** soothes and heals the gastrointestinal mucosa.

14. **Glutathione, L-cysteine, and N-acetylcysteine** provide fuel and act as protective antioxidants and detoxification supporters for the GI mucosa and cellular enzyme systems.

15. **Fiber,** especially the soluble type, such as pectins and gels from fruits and vegetables, protects and promotes proper movement of feces through the GI tract without irritation. Insoluble fiber may also help lessen gut toxicity.

16. **FOS (fructooligosaccharides)** fuels colon bacteria and protects colon cells from pathogenic infections. Some yeast and bacterial strains use FOS as a food source; therefore, it is important to remove or reduce these microbial populations before adding FOS.

17. **Calories** from fresh fruits and vegetables, whole grains, seeds, and legumes are needed to repair damaged or inflamed tissues and maintain energy levels during the GI tract healing program.

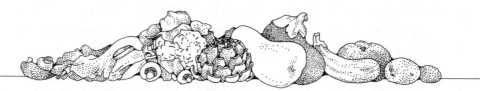

IMPORTANT ELEMENTS OF HEALTHY EATING

- **Eat whole foods,** particularly fresh fruits, vegetables, whole grains, and vegetable proteins (beans, peas, lentils, nuts, and seeds).

- **We are what we eat.** Put only quality food into your body. **Reduce refined foods,** sugar, excess fatty and rich foods, and foods with additives or synthetic coloring. **Avoid** genetically engineered foods and those with chemical herbicides and pesticides by buying foods labeled "organic."

- **Drink** no more than 4 oz of liquids with meals, as it can dilute the digestive juices.

- **Drink 6 to 8 glasses of water daily,** plus herbal teas. Drink 2 to 3 glasses first in the morning and then 1 to 2 glasses an hour or so before lunch and dinner.

- CHEW YOUR FOOD THOROUGHLY, EAT IN A RELAXED ENVIRONMENT, AND RELAX YOURSELF TO PREPARE YOUR BODY FOR NOURISHMENT.

- **Get sufficient fiber** in your diet by eating the majority of your foods from the first tip above and/or by taking additional psyllium seed husks and flaxseed meal.

- Use **nutritional supplements** and herbs as appropriate. Supplement your digestive function as needed with hydrochloric acid, digestive enzymes, and pancreatic products.

- **Moderate** your use of alcohol, caffeine, and nicotine. Beware of excessive use of prescription, OTC, and recreational drugs.

- **Exercise.** If you don't yet have an exercise program, set one up. Do it regularly and with the right combination of activities that will provide strength, flexibility, endurance, and enjoyment.

- **Maintain** regular elimination. Your diet, exercise, and stress levels should allow your bowels to move at least once or twice daily. After illness or antibiotic use, replace friendly GI flora by taking probiotics (acidophilus and other positive digestive bacteria). If this is not sufficient to restore normal digestion and elimination, and your GI function stays irregular for more than a few weeks, seek the advice of a health-care practitioner.

CHAPTER TWO

General Detoxification and Cleansing

◆

Toxicity has become a great concern in our modern world. Threatening our health are powerful chemicals, air and water pollution, radiation, and nuclear waste. We ingest new chemicals, use more drugs, eat more sugary and refined foods, and abuse ourselves daily with stimulants and/or sedatives. Cancer and cardiovascular disease are on the rise; arthritis, allergies, obesity, and skin problems are also rapidly increasing; and a wide range of symptoms such as headaches, fatigue, pains, coughs, gastrointestinal problems, immune weaknesses, sexual diseases, and psychological distress are being seen by physicians in record numbers. Although a connection between increased toxicity and increases in diseases is obvious, it is important to understand how it occurs so that we may avoid or eliminate it from our lives.

Toxicity occurs on two basic bodily levels—external and internal. We can acquire toxins from our environment by breathing them, by ingesting them, or by being in physical contact with them. Most drugs, food additives, and allergens can create toxic elements in the body. In fact, any substance can become toxic when used in excess.

Internally, our body produces toxins through normal everyday functions. Biochemical and cellular activities generate substances that need to be eliminated. These unstable molecules, called *free radicals,* are biochemical toxins and are considered a common factor in chronic disease. When these biochemical toxins are not counteracted or eliminated, they can irritate or inflame the cells and tissues, blocking normal functions on all levels of the body. Microbes such as intestinal bacteria, foreign bacteria, yeasts, and parasites produce metabolic waste products that we must handle. Even our thoughts, emotions, and stress can increase biochemical toxicity. The proper elimination of these toxins is essential. Clearly, the healthy human body can handle certain levels of toxins; **the concern is with excess intake, excess production of toxins, or a reduction in the elimination processes.**

A toxin is basically any substance that creates irritating and/or harmful effects in the body, undermining our health and stressing our biochemical or organ functions.

This irritation may result from the side effects of pharmaceutical drugs or from unusual physiological patterns. The irritating chemicals or free radicals in recreational drugs can also cause tissue degeneration. Negative "ethers," psychic or spiritual influences, bad relationships, thought patterns, and emotions can also have toxic effects on our body.

Toxicity occurs when we ingest more than we can utilize and eliminate. Homeostasis refers to balanced bodily functions. This balance is disturbed when we feed ourselves more than we need or when we abuse specific substances. Toxicity may depend on the dosage, frequency, or potency of the toxin. A toxin may produce an immediate or rapid onset of symptoms, as many pesticides and some drugs do, or it may have long-term effects, as when asbestos exposure leads to lung cancer.

When our body is working well, with good immune and eliminative functions, it can handle everyday exposure to toxins. The purpose of this chapter is to understand the importance of detoxification and to discuss ways to support the elimination of excessive toxins, mucus, congestion, and disease and to prevent the buildup of further toxicity. The cleansing process encourages our immune system to handle the elimination of toxins and abnormal cells generated by the body.

OUR GENERAL DETOXIFICATION SYSTEMS

Gastrointestinal—liver, gallbladder, colon, and the whole GI tract

Urinary—kidneys, bladder, and urethra

Respiratory—lungs, bronchial tubes, throat, sinuses, and nose

Lymphatic—lymph channels and lymph nodes

Skin and dermal—sweat and sebaceous glands and tears

Our body handles toxins either by neutralizing, transforming, or eliminating them. For example, many of the antioxidant nutrients, such as vitamins C and E, beta-carotene, zinc, and selenium may neutralize free-radical molecules. The liver helps transform many toxic substances into harmless agents that the blood carries away to the kidneys; the liver also sends wastes through the bile into the intestines, where they are eliminated. We also clear toxins by sweating, either from exercise or heat; our sinuses expel excess mucus when congested; and our skin releases toxins daily, which can also cause reactions that we may experience as skin rashes.

Mental detoxification is also important. Cleansing our minds of negative thought patterns is essential to health, and physical detoxification can aid this process. Emotionally, detoxification helps us uncover and express hidden frustrations, anger, resentments, and fear, and replace them with forgiveness, love, joy, and hope. Many people experience new clarity of purpose in life during cleansing processes. A light detoxification over a couple of days can help us feel better; a longer process and deeper commitment to eliminating certain abusive habits and eating a better diet can help us change our whole life. Detoxification is part of a transformational medicine that instills change at many levels. Change and evolution are keys to healing.

An important topic to consider in *The New Detox Diet* is electromagnetic toxicity, which has become so commonplace in these modern times with our daily exposure to computers, cell phones, and televisions, plus radiation exposure from airplane travel and medical testing. In some ways, this persistent electrical interaction with our bodies may alter our sensitive cellular, biochemical, immune, and neurological systems. Our bodies are electric (electromagnetic) and clearly our cells and nerves function and communicate electrically. It makes sense that our bodies pick up and can be altered by this interaction. Thus, in addressing toxicity and detoxification, we should be aware of these electromagnetic issues as well.

WHO SHOULD DETOXIFY?

Almost everyone needs to detox and rest their body from time to time. Some of us need to cleanse more frequently or work more continually to rebalance our body. *Cleansing or detoxification* is but one part of the *trilogy of nutritional action* (the others being *building* or *toning,* and *balancing* or *maintenance*). A regular, balanced diet devoid of

Excess Detox? I want to express some concerns about overelimination or overdetoxification, which I occasionally see. Some people go to extremes with fasting, laxatives, enemas, colonics, diuretics, and even exercise, and begin to lose essential nutrients from their body. This can cause protein or vitamin-mineral deficiencies. So, although congestion from overintake and underelimination is a more common problem in this culture, excessive detoxification can be equally harmful.

excess necessitates less intensive detoxification. Our body has a daily elimination cycle, mostly carried out at night and in the early morning up until breakfast. When we eat a congesting diet higher in fats, meats, dairy products, refined foods, and chemicals, detoxification becomes more important, particularly to those who eat excessively, and to those who eat excessively at night.

Our individual lifestyle provides clues for deciding how and when to detoxify. If we have any symptoms or diseases of toxicity and congestion, we will likely benefit more from detoxification practices. It is like a vacation for our body and digestive tract.

Common toxicity symptoms include headache, fatigue, congestion, backaches, aching or swollen joints, digestive problems, "allergy" symptoms, and sensitivity to environmental agents such as chemicals, perfumes, and synthetics. Dietary changes or avoidance of the symptom-causing agents is usually beneficial. However, it is important to differentiate between allergic and toxicity symptoms in order to determine the appropriate medical care. This detox program, as well as fasting and juice cleansing, can all be genuinely helpful in reducing allergy symptoms; however, allergies present a dynamic subtly different from toxicity. The key is to figure out and avoid the allergens from our environment and from our foods. **The detox diet plans in this book will help avoid almost all of the typical allergens we get from our foods and habits.**

SIGNS AND SYMPTOMS OF TOXICITY

Headaches	Frequent colds*	Mood changes*
Joint pains	Irritated eyes	Anxiety
Coughs	Immune weakness*	Depression*
Wheezing	Environmental sensitivity	Sexual dysfunction*
Sore throat	Sinus congestion	Fatigue*
Tight or stiff neck	Fever	Skin rashes*
Angina pectoris	Runny nose	Hives
Circulatory deficits	Nervousness	Nausea
High blood fats	Sleepiness*	Indigestion
Backaches	Insomnia*	Anorexia
Itchy nose	Dizziness*	Bad breath
		Constipation

* These symptoms could also result from deficiency.

Detoxification and cleansing can contribute to the healing of many acute and chronic illnesses that result from short- or long-term congestive patterns. Detox and cleansing benefits people with addictions to numerous substances. However, because **withdrawal symptoms can commonly occur with the detoxification of many drugs, I recommend conscious, informed management of the detox process.**

Detoxification is also an important component in treating obesity. Many of the toxins we ingest or make are stored in the fatty tissues; hence, **obesity is almost always associated with toxicity.** When we lose weight, we reduce our body fat and thereby our toxic load. However, during weight loss we also release more toxins and need to protect ourselves from nutrient depletion through extra supplementation, including taking additional antioxidants to balance these toxins. Exercise will also promote the loss of excess pounds and help further detoxification.

PROBLEMS RELATED TO CONGESTION / STAGNATION / TOXICITY

Acne	Gout	Stroke
Abscesses	Obesity	Prostate disease
Boils	Infections by:	Menstrual problems
Eczema	Bacteria	Vaginitis
Allergies	Virus	Varicose veins
Arthritis	Fungus	Diabetes
Asthma	Parasites	Peptic ulcers
Constipation	Worms	Gastritis
Colitis	Uterine fibroid tumors	Pancreatitis
Hemorrhoids	Cancer	Mental illness
Diverticulitis	Cataracts	Multiple sclerosis
Cirrhosis	Colds	Alzheimer's disease
Hepatitis	Bronchitis	Senility
Fibrocystic breast disease	Pneumonia	Parkinson's disease
Atherosclerosis	Sinusitis	Drug addiction
Heart disease	Emphysema	Tension headaches
Hypertension	Kidney stones	Migraine headaches
Thrombophlebitis	Kidney disease	Gallstones
		Sexual dysfunction

Case Study: Carolyn's Story
Married, Mother, and Businesswoman, age 52

I have been fighting the weight loss game for forty years, always with conventional and not so conventional diets, from Weight Watchers to pills to "fad of the day" diets, and always with the same results. I would lose twenty pounds and gain back forty. By the time the year 2000 came along I was weighing in at 265 lb., and for my height of 5' 7" that was a lot. I decided to go to the Preventive Medical Center of Marin with my husband where Dr. Haas was conducting a group on something called "The Purification Process." I figured, "What have I got to lose?" (Ha!) At the first meeting we discussed the different levels of changing my habits and getting the results that all overweight or unhealthy people seek—long-term weight loss and feeling and being healthier. Our group was embarking on Dr. Haas' Autumn 3-week group program. I first cleaned up my sugar and caffeine habits, the basis of the Detox Diet. Then, onto the False Fat reactive foods, like getting off cow's milk and wheat products. We would even include fasting, the more extreme part of the process, and since I had done that many years before, I thought why not! This whole process worked for me and I started to lose (let go) weight and the feeling of heaviness. I also felt light and more alive. The first couple of days of the fasting part were hard, but I stuck with the Master Cleanser Lemonade (page 61), and all the water, oh, the water.

For the first time I learned what detoxifying really meant. I got off my usual three to four soft drinks a day habit along with all the junk food I had been consuming for years. You could say I was a junk-food junkie. I continued the fast for nine days, and I really could not believe how good I was feeling. The aches and pains I usually had in my legs at bedtime were gone, I was thinking more clearly, and, most important, I was losing weight. For years, I had been taking medication for hypertension, which I assumed I would be on for life. However, that life was changing. With Dr. Haas's guidance and support, I began to decrease my dosage and eventually went off my meds as my blood pressure kept staying low. It's now several years later, and I have not needed to take any medicine since shortly after starting the detox program.

After the fasting, I went on the False Fat Diet (Ballantine Books) more long term and stayed off the sugar, wheat, dairy, and junk foods. I followed The Detox Diet book as well, and to this day, I make this my lifestyle.

From this new way of eating (and I still enjoy my foods, maybe even more as I know I am really nourishing myself), it has been about two years and I have lost a total of ninety pounds. I exercise five days a week, which is something I had not done for more than twenty-five years. I have never felt better, and my skin has improved tremendously. I have a retail jewelry business, and my long-time customers come in and ask me, "Where is the lady that used to work here?" They clearly don't recognize me, or the new me, and that makes me feel great.

I continue to this day to stay free of the sensitive seven foods (wheat, cow's milk, soy, sugar, corn, eggs, and peanuts) and detox two to three times a year. And I have the tools to rebalance myself just in case I do mess up or go off my diet for a day or two. Then I take a few days to get back into my program and feel better again almost immediately. I am completely off any medications and take only supplements. And most important, I continue to love living life.

CASE STUDY: CINDY'S PERSONAL EXPERIENCE
Nurse, age 44

I have PAT (paroxysmal atrial tachycardia), which is when my heart suddenly beats very fast, about two hundred beats per minute. My cardiologist recommended a procedure called a cardiac ablation where they locate the irritable heart cells and destroy them with electrical impulses. It is an invasive surgery and very expensive. I was very scared.

I started to investigate all my options. I was motivated to change my diet and my lifestyle. I knew that the gradual weight gain of fifty pounds over five years was not helping my heart, so I tried many diets. I have been a nurse for twenty-four years so I felt empowered to make better choices in my life so I can live a strong, happy life without this surgery.

I stopped all caffeine, got my cholesterol down to 185 from 210, and did lots of stress management like yoga, energy work, and chanting. I felt better, but the arrthymias continued. I thought I was doing it all right. I was doing my best. I was still working full time as a nurse and was getting more and more frustrated.

I tried so many diets. I was drinking fresh-squeezed carrot juice every day. I was unable to get the weight off. I started to blame myself. I felt like such a failure. I knew that something was missing. That's when I met Dr. Elson Haas.

At our first appointment I told him about my heart and my weight. He said very boldly, "From everything you've told me, I think you have a candida (yeast) problem." I replied, "No, I don't think so. I work full time and am not a chronic fatigue-type person." He asked, "Do you have bloating after your meals?" I said "Yes." He said, "If we can clear you of the Candida, your heart may work better by lowering the yeast toxins in the blood. Let's have you send off blood and stool tests."

Three weeks later I was stunned to learn that I had 4+ *Candida albicans* (that's maximum) growing in my intestines and elevated antibodies in my blood suggesting immune reactivity. He told me to read Chapters One, Two, and Three in his very straightforward book, *The Detox Diet*. He gave me a list of supplements to start on and a sheet on how to do the anti-Candida diet. He had explained how all my good intentions of drinking carrot juice were just like feeding sugar to the yeast. I was encouraged because now we had found a possible culprit. I now knew where to put my energy. Yet still, I didn't know what results to expect.

Within two weeks of following Dr. Haas's recommendations I had lost ten pounds, and I felt great. By ten months I lost a total of forty-eight pounds. Now my heart is regular and strong. My emotional health is so much better. I met the man of my life and at age forty-five I got married for the first time. My PMS is so much less severe, and we are enjoying trying to get pregnant.

I am grateful to Dr. Haas for his precise diagnosis. His wisdom and ability to integrate new ideas into his medical practice truly makes him a pioneer in the health-care field. He found the one piece of the puzzle no one else cared to find. Instead of blaming myself, I was able to clear the yeast from my body, and this made a huge difference. Plus, I made very positive changes in my diet, and this has provided other benefits in terms of better energy, stable moods, and quality sleep. The lifestyle changes took some getting used to, but the hard work paid off.

Today I have been able to tolerate foods I used to be sensitive to, within moderation. And when I do feel bloated or gain weight I am able to go right back on my "program" and feel better.

Of course, not all of these problems are related solely to toxicity, nor will they be completely cured by detoxification. Still, many conditions are created by nutritional abuses and can be alleviated by eliminating the related toxins and following this program.

WHAT IS DETOXIFICATION?

Detoxification is the process of either clearing toxins from the body or neutralizing or transforming them, and hence clearing excess acidity, mucus, and congestion. Fats (especially oxidized fats and cholesterol), free radicals, and other irritating molecules act as toxins on an internal level. Functionally, poor digestion, colon sluggishness and dysfunction, reduced liver function, and poor elimination through the kidneys, respiratory tract, and skin all increase toxicity.

Detoxification involves dietary and lifestyle changes that reduce the intake of toxins while improving elimination. The avoidance of chemicals from food or other sources, including refined flour and sugar products (so plentiful everywhere), caffeine, alcohol, tobacco, and drugs, helps minimize the toxin load. Drinking extra water (purified) and increasing fiber by including more fruits and vegetables in the diet are also essential steps.

A more **rigorous detox diet** is one made up exclusively of fresh fruits, fresh vegetables (either raw or cooked), and whole grains (both cooked and sprouted), plus some raw seeds or sprouted seeds or legumes eaten fresh in salads. No breads or baked goods, animal foods or dairy products, alcohol or nuts are used. This diet keeps fiber and water intake up and hence helps colon detoxification. Most people can handle this quite easily and make the shift from their regular diet with only a few days of transition. Others prefer a **brown rice fast** (a more macrobiotic approach) for a week or two, eating three to four bowls of rice daily along with liquids such as green or herbal teas. Vegetable and miso soups can also be consumed.

An even deeper level of detoxification involves a diet consisting solely of fruits and vegetables—all cleansing foods. The green vegetables, especially the chlorophyllic and high-nutrient leafy greens, support purification of the gastrointestinal tract.

A **raw foods diet** is fulfilling for many people, yielding high energy and quality nutrition. It utilizes sprouted greens from seeds and grains such as wheat, buckwheat, sunflower, alfalfa, and clover; sprouted beans such as mung or garbanzo; soaked or sprouted raw nuts; and fresh fruits and vegetables. Cooked food is not allowed with this diet, as eating foods raw maintains the highest concentrations of vitamins, minerals, and important enzymes. Many people feel that this is their best diet, and I think it can be supportive over quite some time if it is properly balanced.

Detox-healing diets are also available, specifically for problems such as yeast overgrowth or food allergies. In Chapter 5, we include an anti-yeast diet and an anti-allergy (hypoallergenic) diet. They involve aspects of detoxification and re-balance.

The liquid cleanses or fasts move beyond the alkaline detoxification and fruit-and-vegetable diets. Juices, vegetable broths, and teas can be used to purify our body during fasting. Miso soup, made from a paste of fermented soybean, also provides many nutrients and supports colon function by aiding the intestinal bacteria. Spirulina (an algae powder) or other blue-green fresh water algaes can also be helpful to fasters who experience fatigue by providing amino acids for protein building (add to juices for best flavor).

Water fasting is more intense than fasting with juices and often results in more sickness and less energy. Paavo Airola, one of the pioneers of fasting in America, states in *How to Get Well* that "Systematic undereating and periodic fasting are the two most important health and longevity factors." Consuming fresh, diluted juices from various fruits and vegetables can be a safe and helpful approach for many conditions. Furthermore, specific juice regimens may be used beneficially by people for whom water fasts are contraindicated. Juices help to eliminate wastes and dead cells while building new tissue with the easily accessible nutrients. See more in Chapter 3.

The key to proper treatment is to individualize your program. Take into consideration your general health, physiological balance, energy level, and current lifestyle in order to set up the right program for you. **If you are unsure, start with the basic diet**

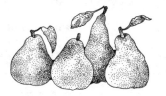

and gradually intensify toward juice fasting and see how you feel. Take a couple of days for each step, and, if you feel fine, move to the next level as described here:

LEVELS OF DIETARY DETOXIFICATION

- Basic Diet
- Reduce Toxins Daily: ingest fewer congesting foods and more nourishing ones (see chart below); for example, decrease drugs, sugar, fried foods, meats, dairy, etc. Eat more fresh fruits and vegetables. Take one to seven days.
- Fruits, vegatables, whole grains, seeds, and legumes
- Raw foods
- Fruits and vegetables
- Fruit and vegetable juices
- Specific juice diets, master cleanser, apple, carrot, and greens, and so on (see Chapter 3: Fasting and Juice Cleansing)
- Water

Detoxification therapy—particularly fasting—is the oldest known medical treatment on Earth and a completely natural process. Of the thousands of people we have worked with who have used cleansing programs, the majority have experienced very positive results. We believe this detoxification process to be a practical and effective health-care therapy in the twenty-first century and an important first step toward healing our planet.

DETOXIFICATION RANGE

Most Congesting ←————————   ————————→ *Least Congesting*

drugs	fats	sweets	nuts	rice	roots	fruits
allergenic foods	fried foods	milk	seeds	millet	squashes	greens herbs
organ meats	refined flour	eggs	beans	buckwheat	other vegetables	water
hydrogenated fats	meats	baked goods	oats	pasta		
			wheat	potatoes		

More Potentially Toxic ←————   ————→ *More Detoxifying*
More Acidic* (generally) ←————   ————→ *More Alkaline**

*The above chart is not exactly acid-alkaline, but suggests a general tendency for the foods and substances on the left to be more acidic, and toward the right, more alkaline.

Ranges of Detoxification

Moving to a less congesting diet, as shown in the facing table, will also induce healing.

The effects of dietary detoxification vary. Even mild changes from our current eating plan will produce some responses, while more dramatic dietary shifts can produce a profound cleansing. Shifting from the most congesting foods to the least—eating more fruits, vegetables, grains, nuts, and legumes and less baked goods, sweets, refined foods, fried foods, and fatty foods—will help most of us detoxify somewhat and bring us into better balance overall.

Maintaining the same diet but adding certain supplements such as fiber, vitamin C, other antioxidants, chlorophyll, and glutathione (mainly as amino acid L-cysteine) can also stimulate detoxification. Herbs such as garlic, red clover, echinacea, or cayenne may also enhance detoxification, as can saunas, sweats, and niacin therapy (see Chapter 6 for more discussion of Supplements for Detoxification). **Simply increasing liquid intake and decreasing fats and refined flour and sugar products will improve elimination and lessen toxin buildup.** Increased consumption of filtered water, herb teas, fruits, and vegetables while reducing fats (especially fried foods, red meat, and milk products) will also help detoxification. A vegetarian diet may also be a healthful step for those with some congestive problems. Meats, milk products, breads, and baked goods (especially refined sugar and carbohydrate products) increase body acidity and lead to more mucus production as the body attempts to balance its chemistry. The more alkaline vegetarian foods enhance cleansing. *The right balance of acid and alkaline foods for each of us is, of course, the key.* *

Acid-Alkaline—A Key to Health and Longevity

The concepts of congestion/toxicity and deficiency/depletion relate to the duality of balance that also includes the acid-alkaline poles. The general ideas about illness and health that are expressed in this book relate to the relative states of acidity, and the congestion, irritation, and inflammation that come from this acid imbalance. The acidity in the body tissues arises from the overintake of too many acid-causing foods (see chart on the facing page). This acidity causes the breakdown and degeneration of tissues over time. **The Detox Diet of steamed vegetables and fresh fruits, water, and**

---

* See Chapters 10 and 12 of *Staying Healthy with Nutrition* for more information on acid and alkaline.

alkaline drinks helps to better balance the body and decrease these acid wastes. The body then lowers its inflammatory and pain states and begins to feel better, more flexible, and more youthful.

The acid-alkaline balance is crucial to what scientists call the "biological terrain" of the body, or the state of the body's tissues and functions. I believe it is this terrain that affects whether or not we are healthy. Parasitic, fungal, and other infections are secondary to imbalances of the terrain; diet, stress levels, and other aspects of lifestyle can profoundly influence the terrain. Since animal products, refined foods (sugars and flours), nuts, and seeds are more acidic in their chemical makeup, they create acid residues when metabolized in the body. They contain higher amounts of the minerals phosphorus, sulfur, chlorine, and iodine, while the more alkaline-generating foods contain higher levels of calcium, magnesium, potassium, and sodium. These include most high-water-content fruits and vegetables, as well as some grains and almonds.

Over time, the consumption of an animal product-based diet creates an acidic state of the tissues, with chronic toxicity shown through congestions, irritation, inflammation, and degeneration. The results of this process are the many painful and terminal diseases people experience as they age.

Over the years I have had patients follow their own pH, or acid, levels—assessing their blood, urine, and saliva, and then monitoring any changes, especially in urine and saliva—to chart their course of healing. There is clearly a strong correlation between body fluid pH and the level of health or disease of the individual. If our tissues accumulate more acid, the kidneys attempt to release acid and withhold bicarbonate, which makes the blood more alkaline.

Acid states appear in people with acute and chronic inflammatory and pain syndromes, congestive disorders that include recurrent infections and allergies, and the degenerative diseases such as cancer, cardiovascular problems, and diabetes. Once these chronic degenerative diseases have set in, they are more difficult to treat or correct. When I have been able to assess and rebalance an individual's biochemistry, I have seen the lessening of symptoms, the halt of disease progression, and even the reversal of some conditions—and I have experienced this with thousands of patients.

And now **The Detox Diet**, originally referred to by me as the Alkaline Detoxification Diet, provides or is a smooth and long-range transitional healing program, many people and problems. It is the great biochemical balancer for the person consuming the typical Western diet, a diet that I have worked diligently to change both personally and professionally, to educate my patients about diet.

CASE STUDY: MARION M

In mid-December of 2002, I had a bad case of the flu and pneumonia. By the end of the month my head and chest symptoms had cleared up. But I was weak and had a slight stomachache most of the time; my stools looked different. Since I had not seen a doctor in two years, I found an internist who prescribed a battery of tests, including my blood, urine, a mammogram, an ultrasound, and a bone density test. The last revealed some osteoporosis while the rest of my tests turned out fairly normal. Then I went to a gastroenterologist who did scopes and biopsies, which revealed celiac sprue (an inability to tolerate wheat and other gluten grains). It was suggested that I follow a gluten-free eating plan for the rest of my life, avoiding all wheat products, as well as rye, barley, and oats.

I joined the Houston Celiac Support Group, and became totally dedicated to my gluten-free way of life, going so far as never licking envelopes, as the glue might contain wheat, and just throwing out my lotions that might have oats in them. However, I was still losing weight with accompanying problems such as extreme weakness, depression, sores in my mouth, leg cramps, some joint soreness, and weakened eyesight. I was so thin that my exposed bones made it very uncomfortable to sit on any hard surface. It was also very upsetting to look at myself in the mirror and see an old, wrinkled woman.

Diarrhea alternating with constipation continued, but I was so steeped in the celiac philosophy that I actually had thought I was improving. On the GF (gluten-free) eating program, my husband and I decided I was strong enough to go to Sun Valley, but before going, I had called a friend to inquire about finding a dietitian in the area to help me. That's how I came to know Daniella Chace. She suggested I have my doctor run a food allergy (antibody) test and some stool tests to see if my gut had something to do with feeling so poorly. The blood testing revealed a list of temporary food reactions, but also had a long list of safe foods, including gluten, my supposed archenemy.

What was I to do with this news and my supposed Celiac disease? I waited another week for my stool test results, and then Daniella called to tell me that I had giardiasis, a giardia infection! I excitedly called my internist, who prescribed metronidazole, a strong antiparasitic drug I was to take over seven days. I had forgotten to get my endoscopy results. My internist faxed me the report, which concluded, "The structures are histologically compatible with giardia."

Why had no one contacted me about this? My case had fallen through the cracks in Houston, the home of the famous Texas Medical Center. It had taken an alert, cutting-edge nutritionist in a small Idaho town to properly diagnose me. I feel that Daniella Chace literally saved my life, at least the quality. She also put me on an eating program of healthful supplements to repair my damaged intestines and had scheduled a gradual intake of the foods as all my allergies seemed to disappear. After three months of this good regimen, plus one and a half hours of exercise daily, I'm now in the best shape ever. I am still on Daniella's supplement program, and I continue to heal. I am now thoroughly convinced that nutritionists and other naturally oriented practitioners should be playing a greater role in our lives.

CASE STUDY: TOBIN J
Cameraman, age 30

Tobin lives in Sun Valley, Idaho, and came to one of my (Daniella's) Spring Detox classes in hopes to regain energy and vitality. He came away with some unexpected results.

He cleaned the toxins from his home and eliminated chemicals and toxic foods from his diet. Tobin explained, "I was surprised to find that as my body became cleaner, my mind became clear, and I no longer tolerated emotional frustrations. I felt like I had to rid myself of "toxic emotions." He went to the extent of facing up to his boss and expressing some long repressed feelings.

Tobin also felt that the cleansing work he did and the fast acted as a catalyst that helped him clarify his relationship with food. "I was eating when I wasn't even hungry. I saw this clearly. I had been feeding my inner child junk food as a treat and now I see that emotional process going on and I can intervene. I did intervene."

WHEN IS THE BEST TIME TO DETOXIFY?

Whenever we feel congested, our first step is to follow detoxification procedures fine-tuned to our specific needs. When we start to feel congested from too much food, people, or activities, we will feel better if we can exercise, sauna or steam, drink loads of fluids, eat lightly, take vitamins C and A, and get a good night's sleep. If you feel like your colon requires further cleansing, take stimulating, laxative-type herbs.

Our bodies have natural cleansing cycles when they want a lighter diet, more liquids, and greater elimination than intake. This occurs daily (usually from the night until midmorning, about an hour after we wake) and it may occur for longer periods weekly and more commonly for a few days a month. Women, in particular, are aware of this natural cleansing time with their menstrual cycle. In fact, many women feel better both premenstrually and during their periods if they follow a simple cleansing program of more juices, greens, lighter foods, and herbs during or around their menses.

In the yearly cycle, *seasonal changes* are key times of stress when we may need to *reduce our outer demands and consumptions* and listen to the way our inner world mirrors the natural events.* **Spring and autumn are good times for yearly detoxification.**

---

* To gain a more healthful understanding of your seasonal cycles, see my book *Staying Healthy with the Seasons*.

I suggest at least a one- to two-week program at these times. In spring, we may eat more citrus fruits, fresh greens, juices, or the **Master Cleanser lemonade diet** (see page 61); while in autumn we may dine on harvest fruits, such as apples or grapes, and seasonal vegetables. An abundance of fresh fruits and vegetables are appropriate for summer; and whole grains, legumes, vegetables, and soups best simplify our diet in winter.

The sample yearly program provided here is designed for a basically healthy person who eats well. It is not appropriate for people with heart problems, extreme fatigue, underweight conditions, or poor circulation (those who experience coldness). More complete, in-depth fasting programs may release even greater amounts of toxins (see Chapter 3: Fasting and Juice Cleansing). **Releasing too much toxicity can make sick people sicker; if this happens, increase fluids and eat normally again until you feel better.** People with cancer need to be very careful about how they detoxify, and often they need regular, quality nourishment.

Note: Fasting should be done only under the care of an experienced physician (usually one that is naturopathically trained and that could be M.D.s, D.O.s, N.D.s, D.C.s, and more). All people should avoid fasting just prior to surgery and wait four to six weeks before fasting or any strenuous detoxifying. Pregnant or lactating women should avoid heavy detoxification, though they can usually handle mild programs, which should be undertaken only with the guidance of a qualified practitioner.

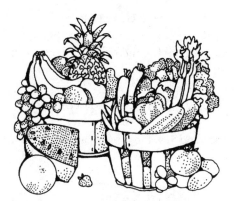

SAMPLE YEAR-LONG DETOX PROGRAM

Note for Detox: When buying your fruits and vegetables, look for organic, seasonal, and fresh whenever possible.

~ SPRING ~

For 7–21 days between March 10 and April 15 (or later in the cold or in the northern climates) use one or more of the following plans:

- Master Cleanser (lemonade diet, see p. 61).
- Fruits, vegetables, and leafy greens, including blue-green algaes (spirulina, chlorella, and blue-green algae).
- Juices of fruits, vegetables, and greens.
- Herbs with any of the above.
- These plans can be alternated or can include a 3–5 day supervised water fast.
- Remember to take time for the transition back to the regular diet (about half as long as the fast itself), which hopefully will have changed for the better.
- Elimination and food testing can also be done at this time.

(see Recipes in Chapters 4 and 13)

~ MID-SPRING ~

Take a 3-day cleanse around mid-May as a reminder of healthy habits and as an enhancer of food awareness.

~ SUMMER ~

Try one week of fruits and vegetables and/or fresh juices to usher in the warm weather sometime between June 10 and July 4.

~ LATE SUMMER ~

Take a 3-day cleanse of fruit and vegetable juices around mid- to late August.

~ Autumn ~

Take a 7–10 day cleanse between September 11 and October 5, such as:

- Grape fast—whole and juiced—all fresh and preferably organic.
- Apple and lemon juice together, diluted.
- Fresh fruits and vegetables, raw and cooked.
- Fruit and vegetable juices—fruit in the morning, vegetables in the afternoon.
- Juices plus spirulina, algae, or other green chlorophyll powders.
- Whole grains, cooked squashes, and other vegetables (a lighter detox).
- Mixture of the above plans, with garlic as a prime detoxifier.
- Basic low-toxicity diet, with additional herbal program.
- Colon detox with fiber (psyllium, pectin, etc.) along with enemas or colonics.
- Prepare and plan a new autumn diet, enhancing positive dietary habits.

~ Mid-Autumn ~

Take a 3-day cleanse with juices or in-season produce in late October to early November.

~ Winter ~

A lighter diet, eaten for a week or two in preparation for the holidays (or as detox from them) can be done between December 10 and January 5:

- Avoid toxins and treats; eat a very basic wholesome diet.
- One week of brown rice, cooked vegetables, miso broth, and seaweed. Ginger and cayenne pepper can be used in soups.
- Saunas or steams and massage—you deserve it!
- Hang on until spring!

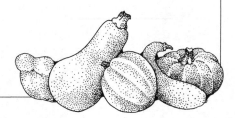

WHERE CAN WE DETOXIFY?

During basic, simple detoxification programs, most of us can maintain our normal daily routine. In fact, energy, performance, and health often improve. For some, the detox process may produce headaches, fatigue, irritability, mucous congestions, or aches and pains for the first few days. Any of the symptoms of toxicity may appear, however, usually they don't. Symptoms that have been experienced previously may reoccur transiently during detoxification; sometimes it is hard to know whether or not to treat them. Since my approach to medicine is to allow the body to heal itself, I support the natural healing process whenever possible unless the person is very uncomfortable or the practitioner or patient is very concerned.

It is wise to begin new programs, diets, or lifestyle changes with a few days at home. In time, experience will show what works best. Most of us can maintain a regular work schedule during a cleanse or detox program (and we may even be more productive). However, it might be easier to begin a program on a Friday, as the first few days are usually the hardest. Some of us may be more sensitive during cleansing to the stress of our work environment or to chemical exposures. Also, co-workers or family members may provide temptations or challenge our decisions. Having supportive guides or co-cleansers can be a great comfort and source of positive reinforcement when our inner resolve begins to fade. At the end of the first or second day, usually around dinnertime, symptoms like headache and fatigue may begin to appear, and it is good to be able to rest and spend time in familiar, undemanding surroundings. By the third day, we usually feel pretty stable and ready for work.

Still, many people like to start new programs on a Monday, knowing that they will do fine, using willpower and visualization to see themselves through. People often feel better than ever and are able to accomplish tasks and meet challenges more easily than usual. In fact, experienced fasters may utilize fasting during busy work periods to improve their productivity. Preparing and planning, clearing doubts and fears, and keeping a daily journal are all useful during this vital process and are crucial to any successful undertaking.

WHY DETOXIFY?

We detoxify/cleanse for health, vitality, and rejuvenation—to clear symptoms, treat disease, and prevent future problems. A cleansing program is an ideal way to help us reevaluate our lives, make changes, or clear abuses and addictions. Withdrawal happens fairly rapidly, and as cravings are reduced we can begin a new life without the addictive habits or drugs.

We cleanse because it makes us feel more vital, creative, and open to emotional and spiritual energies. Many people detox/cleanse (or, more commonly, fast on water or juices) for spiritual renewal and to feel more alive, awake, and aware. Jesus Christ, Paramahansa Yogananda, Mahatma Ghandi, Dr. Martin Luther King, Jr., and many other spiritual and religious teachers have advocated fasting for spiritual and physical health. Some celebrities, such as Willie Nelson, practice juice fasting.

Detoxification can be helpful for weight loss, although this is not its primary purpose. Cleansing is more important as an overall lifestyle and dietary transition. However, just the simplification of our diet will have some detoxifying effects in our body. Anyone eating 4,000 calories daily of fatty, sweet foods in a poorly balanced diet who begins to eat 2,000 to 2,500 calories daily of more wholesome foods will definitely experience detoxification, weight loss, and improved health simultaneously.

We also cleanse/detoxify to rest or heal our overloaded digestive organs and allow them to catch up on past work and get current. At the same time, we are inspired to cleanse our external life as well, cleaning out rooms, sorting through the piles on our desks, clarifying our personal priorities, or revitalizing our wardrobes. Most often our energy is increased and becomes steadier, motivating us to change both internally and externally.

REASONS FOR CLEANSING

Prevent disease	Clear skin	Productive
Reduce symptoms	Slow aging	Relaxed
Treat disease	Improve flexibility	Energetic
Cleanse body	Improve fertility	Conscious
Rest organs	Enhance the senses	Inwardly attuned
Purification	**To be more:**	Spiritual
Rejuvenation	Creative	Environmentally attuned
Weight loss	Motivated	Relationship focused

FOOD ADDITIVE CASES

J.B., age 39
When I eat Chinese food seasoned with MSG (monosodium glutamate) I feel pressure on my face. It's like a crushing feeling. It must be pretty poisonous to cause such an immediate and intense reaction.

C.B., age 28
MSG (monosodium glutamate) makes my arms and legs go numb for about an hour after I eat it. I am always careful to let my waiter know that I don't want any MSG in my food when I eat at Chinese restaurants.

G.M., age 55
GM is a successful woman in her fifties who was dealing with anger management and uncontrollable emotions. She kept a diet diary for a few weeks, and Daniella saw that she ate Red Vine candy (corn syrup candy colored with red dye #40) all day long, almost as a nervous habit. She has an addictive personality and finds it hard to have moderate amounts of any substance she's using, whether it is coffee, drugs, alcohol, or sugar. Daniella advised her to stop eating Red Vines with red dye #40, which has been linked to ADHD (attention deficit hyperactivity disorder) and behavioral problems in children, as well as adults. Within days she felt "less irritated" and after a week all angry feelings had subsided. She then felt a long lost feeling of "well-being again."

Food Chemical Exposure

In Daniella's clinical experience, she has found that her client's symptoms are often associated with toxic exposure. Many people come to her office in search of nutrients to relieve their symptoms, such as headaches, joint pain, nervous disorders, infertility, and skin conditions. Yet, what she finds is that they primarily need to eliminate rather than add. Toxic food chemicals are often the culprits. Once they have eliminated or reduced exposure to chemicals, including hormones, food colorings, preservatives, sulfites, pesticides, and herbicides (with organic foods), they experience a marked reduction in symptoms while regaining their health and vitality.

Although we are exposed daily to chemicals through our water, air, cleaning products, and personal care products, our greatest risk of chemical exposure is through our foods. This is also the area over which we have the most control. If you suspect food chemical reactions are a problem for you, try to avoid them by reading labels and buying organic produce, meats, packaged products, and dairy. Also, when eating in restaurants ask them for more organic foods. If we all begin asking and demanding chemical-free foods and products, we will continue to support this growing, necessary organic industry.

Hygiene Awareness

Proper hygiene inside and outside our body and personal environment is one of the four laws of good health, along with eating an alkaline-based diet of wholesome foods, exercising daily, and having proper rest, relaxation, and recreation. Although I believe that germs have a harder time causing problems in a healthy body, they do cause certain kinds of problems from mild colds and flus to life-threatening infections. Therefore, do what you can to protect yourself and do not share your germs too freely with others.

HEALTHY HYGIENE HINTS

1. Wash your hands several times daily—especially after eliminating, before handling food, after handling animals/pets, when you are sick with an upper respiratory problem (coughing, sneezing, or runny nose), or when you are in close physical contact with others. Also, clean up after a public encounter, such as hand-shaking, door-opening, or using public phones.

2. Bathe or shower at least once daily, more if you are sweaty or dirty, in a clean tub or shower; also, use environmentally friendly hygiene products and cleansers.

3. Exercise and sweat regularly to help cleanse your skin and move the lymphatic fluids.

4. Keep your nails clean and cut, and clear out dirt and germs that may get under them with hydrogen peroxide or a nail brush.

5. Do not put used utensils or your hands into group food.

6. Blow your nose and rinse out your nose and sinuses when you are congested.

7. Follow safe sex guidelines, especially with a new partner.

8. Make sure your diet and activity level facilitate at least one to two good bowel movements a day and clean yourself properly afterward.

9. Keep your kitchen and refrigerator clean; wash counters and cutting boards regularly. Don't let germs breed in your trash bins—wash them regularly as well.

10. Minimize your use of and exposure to chemicals at home and in the workplace. Don't replace germs and dirt with chemicals.

CHAPTER THREE

Fasting and Juice Cleansing

Fasting is the single greatest natural healing therapy I know. It is nature's ancient, universal remedy for many problems, used instinctively by animals when ill and by earlier cultures for healing and spiritual purification. When I first discovered fasting over twenty-five years ago, I felt as if it had saved my life. My stagnant energies began flowing, my allergies, aches, and pains disappeared, and I became more creative and vitally alive. I still find fasting both a useful personal tool and an important therapy for many medical and life problems.

Most of the conditions for which fasting is appropriate are ones that result from excess nutrition rather than undernourishment. Dietary abuses generate many chronic degenerative diseases such as atherosclerosis, hypertension, heart disease, allergies, diabetes, cancer, and substance abuse that undermine our health and precede the breakdown of the body. Fasting is not only therapeutic but, more important, acts in preventing many conditions. It often becomes the catalyst for shifting from unhealthy or abusive habits to a more healthful lifestyle in general.

As we use the term here, fasting refers to the avoidance of solid food and the intake of liquids only. True fasting would be the total avoidance of anything by mouth. The most stringent form of fasting allows drinking water exclusively; more liberal fasting includes the juices of fresh fruit and vegetables as well as herbal teas. All of these methods generate a high degree of detoxification—eliminating toxins from the body. Individual experiences with fasting depend upon the overall condition of the body, mind, and attitude. **Detoxification can be intense and may either temporarily increase sickness or be immediately helpful and uplifting.**

Juice fasting is commonly used as an effective cleansing plan. Fresh juices are easily assimilated and require minimum digestion, while still supplying many nutrients and stimulating our body to clear wastes. It is also safer than water fasting as it supports the body nutritionally (at least somewhat) while cleansing and hence maintains bodily energy levels, producing better detoxification and a quicker recovery.

I believe that fasting is the "missing link" in the Western diet and lifestyle. Most people overeat, eat too often, and eat a high-protein, high-fat, acid-congesting diet more consistently than is necessary. If we regularly eat a balanced, well-combined, more "alkalinizing" diet we will have less need for fasting and toning plans (although both are still highly beneficial performed at intervals throughout the year).

Detoxification is a time when we allow our cells and organs to breathe and restore themselves. However, we do not necessarily need to fast to experience some cleansing. Even minor dietary shifts, including an increase in fluids, more raw foods, and fewer congesting foods, will initiate and promote better bodily function and improved detoxification. For example, a vegetarian or macrobiotic diet will be very cleansing and purifying to someone on a heavier diet. The general process of detoxification is discussed thoroughly in Chapter 2: General Detoxification. Here we focus on fluid fasting's history, benefits, and therapeutic use.

Fasting is a time-proven remedy, with human origins going back many thousands of years. Voluntary abstinence from food has been a tradition in most religions and is still used as a spiritual purification rite. Religions such as Christianity, Judaism, Islam, Buddhism, and Hinduism have encouraged fasting as penance, preparation for ceremony, purification, mourning, sacrifice, divine union, and enhancement of mental and spiritual powers. The Bible is filled with stories of people fasting for purification and communion with God. The Essenes, authors of the Dead Sea Scrolls, also advocated fasting as one of their primary methods of healing and spiritual revelation, as described in *The Essene Gospel of Peace* (translated by Edmond Bordeaux Szekely from the third-century Aramaic manuscript).

Philosophers, scientists, and physicians across time have fasted as a means to promote life and health after sickness. Socrates, Plato, Aristotle, Galen, Paracelsus, and Hippocrates all used fasting therapy. Many of today's spiritual teachers also recommend fasting as a useful tool. In a lecture entitled "Healing by God's Unlimited Power" (1947), Paramahansa Yogananda suggested that fasting increased our natural resistance to disease, stating that "Fasting is a natural method of healing. When animals or savages are sick, they fast. Most diseases can be cured by judicious fasting. Unless one has a weak heart, regular short fasts have been recommended by the yogis as an excellent health measure."

Through the centuries, physicians and healers have treated a variety of maladies with fasting, acknowledging that *ignorance of how to live in accordance with nature may be our greatest disease.* Our inherent knowledge of how to live according to the natural laws and spiritual truths leads to the sacred wisdom of life and subsequent good health. Knowing when and how long to fast is part of this knowledge. Through fasting, we can turn our energies inward, where we can use them for healing, clarity, and change.

Physicians with a spiritual orientation tend to be more inclined than others to employ fasting, both personally and in their practices. Many of my own life transitions were stimulated and supported through fasting; when I have felt blocked or needed creative energy in my writing, fasting has been very useful. *In Spiritual Nutrition and the Rainbow Diet,* physician and spiritual teacher Gabriel Cousens, M.D., includes an excellent chapter on fasting in which he describes his theories and his own forty-day regime. According to Dr. Cousens,

". . . fasting in a larger context, means to abstain from that which is toxic to mind, body, and soul. A way to understand this is that fasting is the elimination of physical, emotional, and mental toxins from our organism, rather than simply cutting down on or stopping food intake. Fasting for spiritual purposes usually involves some degree of removal of oneself from worldly responsibilities. It can mean complete silence and social isolation during the fast which can be a great revival to those of us who have been putting our energy outward."

From a medical point of view, fasting is not utilized often enough. We take vacations from work to relax, recharge, and gain new perspectives on our life—why not take occasional breaks from food? (Or, for that matter, from excessive activity or television and communication devices?) To break the habit of eating three meals a day is a challenge for most of us. When we stop and let our stomach remain empty, our body goes into an elimination cycle, and most people will experience some withdrawal symptoms, especially when toxicity exists. Symptoms include headaches, irritability, or fatigue. As with all allergy-addictions, eating again assuages these symptoms.

Fasting is a useful therapy for so many conditions and people. Those who tend to develop congestive symptoms do well with fasting; congestive acidic conditions include colds, flus, bronchitis, mucus congestion, and constipation *(see the long lists of symptoms and medical conditions that may benefit from detoxification in the previous chapter)*. If not addressed, such conditions can lead to headaches, chronic intestinal problems, skin conditions, and more severe ailments. Most of us living in Western, industrialized nations suffer from both overnutrition and undernutrition. We take in excessive amounts of potentially toxic nutrients, such as fats, sugars, and chemicals, and inadequate amounts of many essential vitamins and minerals. The resulting congestive diseases are characterized by excess mucus and sluggish elimination; deficiency problems result from either poor nourishment or ineffective digestion/assimilation. Juice fasting supplies nutrients while still allowing for the elimination of toxins.

Juice fasting/cleansing can be used both to detoxify from drugs and when embarking on a new lifestyle transition, provided there are no contraindications (discussed later in this chapter). Short-term fasting is versatile and generally safe; however, when used to treat medical conditions, proper supervision should be employed. Many physicians, chiropractors, acupuncturists, and nutritionists feel comfortable overseeing people during cleansing/detox programs, and I encourage you to seek them out if your condition warrants supervision. Make sure they're not only theoretical but practical in their own self-knowledge and experience.

Do You Experience Any of These Conditions for Which Fasting May Be Beneficial?		
Colds	Environmental allergies	Diabetes
Flus	Asthma	Fever
Bronchitis	Insomnia	Fatigue
Headaches	Skin conditions	Back pains
Constipation	Atherosclerosis	Mental illness
Indigestion	Coronary artery disease	Obesity
Diarrhea	Angina pectoris	Cancer
Food allergies	Hypertension	Epilepsy

- The use of **fasting** as a treatment for fevers is controversial. It shouldn't be. Consuming liquids generates less heat, and this helps cool the body. With fever, we need more liquids than usual.

- Some cases of **fatigue** respond well to fasting, particularly when the fatigue results from congested organs and stalled energy. With fatigue that results from chronic infection, nutritional deficiency, or serious disease, added nourishment is probably called for as opposed to fasting.

- **Back pain** caused by muscular tightness and stress (rather than from bone disease or osteoporosis) are usually alleviated with a lighter diet or juice fasting. Much tightness and soreness along the back results from colon or other organ congestion; in my experience, poor bowel function and constipation are commonly associated with back pain.

- Patients with **mental illness** ranging from anxiety to schizophrenia may be helped by fasting. Although this may sound sensational, fasting's purpose here, however, is not to cure these problems, but rather to help understand the relationship of foods, chemicals, and drugs with mental functioning. Additional allergies and environmental reactions are not at all uncommon in people with mental illness. True, the release of toxins or lack of nourishment during fasting may worsen psychiatric problems; if, however, the patient is strong and congested, fasting may be helpful. The supervision of a health-care provider is important for patients with mental illness.

- People often attempt to remedy **obesity** by fasting, although it is not the best use of this healing technique. Fasting is actually too temporary an approach for overweight dieters and may even generate feasting reactions in people coming off the fast. A better solution would be a more gradual change of diet with a longer-term weight-reduction plan—something that will replace old dietary habits and food choices with new ones. However, a short 5- to 10-day fast can motivate people to make the necessary dietary changes and renewed commitments to proper eating.

  Some very obese patients who have needed to shed weights of a hundred pounds or more have been on month-long water fasts supervised in hospitals. Other patients have had their jaws wired shut allowing them to only ingest fluids through straws. Still others have surgery to shrink their stomach size. Newer fasting programs substitute a variety of protein-rich powders for meals. These are also usually medically supervised and are for people who are at least thirty to fifty pounds overweight. These pre-packaged, high-protein, low-calorie diets allow patients to burn more fat. Although these programs are not nearly as healthful as vital juice fasts, they are more nutritionally supportive over a longer period of time and can be used on an outpatient basis fairly safely if people are monitored regularly. They provide all the needed vitamins, minerals, and amino acids to sustain life while helping many people lower their weight, blood fats, blood pressure, and blood sugars. However, as with any weight-loss program, success depends upon participant motivation to change personal diets and habits permanently, as fluctuating weights may actually be more harmful than just remaining overweight. Many obese people are also deficient in nutrients because they eat a highly refined, fatty, sweet diet. They are often fatigued and need to be nourished first before they will do well on any fast. A well-balanced, low-calorie, low-chemical (yet high-nutrient) diet with lots of exercise is still the best way to reduce and maintain a good weight and figure.

- Fasting to treat **cancer** is a controversial topic but is used by many alternative clinics outside the United States. Because of cancer's extremely debilitating effects, this may not be wise. Juice fasting may be helpful in the early stages of cancer and is definitely a preventive measure as it reduces toxicity. Anyone with cancer needs adequate nourishment; adding fresh juices to an already wholesome diet can promote mild detoxification and enhance overall vitality. Consult with an experienced practitioner first for individual treatment guidance.

THE PROCESS AND BENEFITS OF FASTING

Although the results of fasting will vary depending upon the individual condition of the faster, there are a number of metabolic changes and experiences that are common to all. First, fasting is a catalyst for change and an essential part of transformational medicine. It promotes relaxation and energization of the body, mind, and emotions, and supports a greater spiritual awareness. Many fasters let go of past experiences and develop a positive attitude toward the present. Having plenty of energy to get things done and cleaning up our personal and community environment are also common responses to the cleansing process. Fasting definitely improves motivation and stimulates creative energy; it also enhances health, beauty, and vitality by letting many of the body systems rest.

Fasting is a multidimensional experience, affecting people physically, mentally, emotionally, and spiritually. Breaking down stored or circulating chemicals is its basic process; the blood and lymph also have the opportunity to be cleaned of toxins as their eliminative functions are alleviated. Each cell has the opportunity to catch up on its work; with fewer new demands, cells can repair themselves and eliminate wastes. Most fasters experience a new vibrancy of their skin and clarity of mind and body. Most important, our liver can spend more time detoxifying our body and creating new essential substances. Two to three quarts of water and juices daily (or even more in some people) are optimal during fasting to cleanse and support the body.

Metabolically, fasting initially reduces caloric intake to the point where the liver converts stored glycogen to glucose and energy. Body fat and fatty acids can be used for energy (ATP); however, the brain and central nervous system need direct glucose. With fasting, some protein breakdown occurs (less if calories are provided by juices). When glycogen stores are low, the body can convert protein to amino acids and to energy—specifically the amino acids alanine and serine can be used to produce glucose. Fatty acids can also be a source of energy during fasting, as they convert to ketones (acetone bodies), which can be used by the body to prevent protein loss. With juice fasting, there is less ketosis (disrupted carbohydrate metabolism), and the simple carbohydrates provided by the juices are easily used for energy and cellular function. High-protein (fasting) diets and other weight-loss programs may burn more fat and generate more ketosis, but they also add more toxins and may create other health concerns.

Fasting increases the process of elimination and the release of toxins from the colon, kidneys, bladder, lungs, sinuses, and skin. This process can generate discharges such as mucus, which helps clear biochemical suffocation. Fasting helps us decrease this suffocation by allowing the cells to eliminate waste products, increase oxygenation, and improve cellular nutrition.

SOME BENEFITS OF FASTING

Purification	Drug detoxification
Rejuvenation	Better resistance to disease
More energy	Spiritual awareness
Rest for digestive organs	More restful sleep
Greater abdominal peace	More relaxation
Clearer skin	Greater motivation and optimism
Sense of personal beauty	New inspiration and creativity
Anti-aging effects	More clarity, mental and emotional
Improved senses—vision, hearing, taste	Improved communications
Self-confidence	Better organization
Reduction of allergies	Clean personal space
Weight loss	Cleaner boundaries for energy in and out
Clothes fit more comfortably	Commitment to habit changes
	Diet changes, long term

As for fasting symptoms, headache is not at all uncommon during the first day or two. Hunger is usually present for two or three days and then departs, leaving many people with a surprising feeling of deep "abdominal peace." When hungry, it is good to ask ourselves, "What are we hungry for?" Fasting is an excellent time to work on the psychological aspects of consumption. Fatigue or irritability may arise at times, as may dizziness or lightheadedness. Sensitivity is usually increased, and common sounds like the telephone, television, music, or the hum of a refrigerator or air-conditioner may be more irritating. Our sense of smell is also exaggerated. Most people's tongues will develop a thick white or yellow fur coating, which can be scraped or brushed off. Bad breath and displeasing tastes in the mouth, or foul-smelling urine or stools, may occur. Skin odor or skin eruptions such as small spots or painful boils may also appear, depending on the level of toxicity. Digestive upset, mucus-containing stools, flatulence, or even nausea and vomiting may also occur. Some people experience insomnia or bad dreams as their body releases poisons during the night. Wild dreams about weird foods are not uncommon. Believe me though, the ultimate benefits are well worth the transient discomforts.

The mind may put up resistance, sending messages of doubt or fear that fasting is not right. This can be exaggerated by listening to other people's fears about your fasting. (If you are looking for excuses not to fast, they are everywhere.) Most symptoms will occur early on (if at all) and will pass. Generally, energy levels are good, although energy may go down every two or three days as the body excretes more wastes. It is at these times that resistance and fears (as well as new symptoms) may arise; if symptoms occur, it is wise to drink more fluids. However, most people will feel cleaner, better, and more alive most of the time.

Old symptoms or patterns from the past may arise during fasts—again usually transiently—or new symptoms of detoxification may appear. This "crisis" or periodic cleansing is not predictable and often raises doubts and questions—is this a new problem or part of the healing process? Generally, time and the healing process will sort things out. We should use Hering's Law of Cure to guide us in making these judgment calls. It states that healing happens from the inside out, the top down, from more important organs to less important ones, and from the most recent to the oldest symptoms. Most healing crises pass within a day or two, although some cleansers experience several days of "cold" symptoms or sinus congestion. If any symptom lasts longer than two or three days, it should be considered a side effect or new problem and should be addressed accordingly. If a problem worsens or causes concern (fainting, heart arrhythmias, or bleeding), the fast should be stopped and a doctor consulted.

Medical supervision is important for anyone in poor health or without fasting experience. If the fast is extended for more than three or four days, regular monitoring, including physical examinations and blood work, should be done weekly (particularly if there is any cause for concern). Fasting may reduce blood protein levels and will definitely lower blood fats. Uric acid levels may rise due to protein breakdown, while levels of some minerals such as potassium, sodium, calcium, or magnesium may drop. Iron levels are usually lower, and the red blood cell count may also drop slightly during this time. Lowered mineral levels can result in fatigue or muscle cramps; if these should occur, additional minerals (particularly calcium, magnesium, and potassium) should be taken, ideally in a powdered form for easy assimilation.

Nutritionally, fasting helps us appreciate the more subtle aspects of our diet, as less food and simple flavors will become more satisfying (even food aromas can be fulfilling). Mentally, fasting improves clarity and attentiveness; emotionally, it may make us more sensitive and aware of our feelings. Individuals may gain the clarity to make important decisions during this therapy. Fasting definitely supports the transformational, evolutionary process. Juice fasting offers a lesson in self-restraint and control of passions. This new and empowering sense of self-discipline can be highly motivating. Fasters who were once spectators suddenly become doers.

CASE STUDY, K.F.
Mother, age 38

I have been a patient of Dr. Haas for many years. He does inspire me to care for myself and my family as well as treat any problems that come up. I know he is always thinking of the safest and most natural way to treat us.

Therefore, when he told me about his detox groups, I elected to participate. I will briefly explain my experiences. I am basically healthy and not really overweight. Yet, I have had knee pains and some arthritis patterns since I was a teenager. And my energy does wax and wane over the month and year. I just couldn't figure out any of the causes.

First I did the three-week Autumn Detox Program with a large group of people. I got off sugar and caffeine, and then in the second week, off wheat, dairy, eggs, and the rest of the Sensitive Seven (sugar, corn, soy, and peanuts). Then, the third week, we started to bring some of these foods back. It was great! Immediately I could tell that wheat and dairy products made me sluggish and congested in my nose and head. And my knees felt better at first, and then the aches and pains came back.

I didn't really connect with this since I had no thought that my twenty years of pain would have any relevance to this process. But, I did feel better overall.

In spring, Dr. Haas motivated me to do his ten-day Spring Cleanse, more of a juice diet. I was open, even though I was concerned about losing weight. However, I did make it through with the other twenty-five people. I felt amazing! And what's more, my knees were totally pain-free for the first time. Now, Dr. Haas encouraged me to come back into my diet slowly, which I was happy to do since I felt so good drinking juices and now eating lightly, mostly fresh fruits and vegetables. As I progressed into other foods, I saw that wheat, dairy, and sugar and corn syrup made my knees ache. It was very cool to connect this and gain power over this chronic pain. I say that because more than a year later, my knees and my body still feel much better. I would never have thought that these simple food reactions could be contributing to this chronic problem. Thank you, Dr. Haas, for this experiential and awakening education.

HAZARDS OF FASTING

If fasting is overused, it may create depletion and weakness in the body, lowering resistance and increasing susceptibility to disease. While fasting does allow the organs, tissues, and cells to rest and handle excesses, the body needs the nourishment provided by food to function after it has used up its stores.

Malnourished people should definitely not fast, nor should some overweight people who are undernourished. Others who should not fast include people with fatigue resulting from nutrient deficiency, those with chronic degenerative disease of the muscles or bones, or those who are underweight. Diseases associated with clogged or toxic organs respond better to fasting. Sluggish individuals who retain water or whose weight is concentrated in their hips and legs often do worse. Those with low daytime energy and more vitality at night (more yin or alkaline types) may not enjoy fasting either.

Fasting is not recommended for pregnant or lactating women, or for people who have weak hearts or weakened immunity. (However, women can use short juice cleanses during their menstrual cycle to help ease pain and other symptoms.) Before or after surgery is not a good time to fast, as the body needs its nourishment to handle the stress and healing demands of the operation. Although some nutritional therapies for cancer include medically supervised fasting, *We do not recommend fasting for cancer patients, particularly those with advanced problems.* Ulcer disease is not something for which fasting is suggested, either, although fasting may be beneficial for other conditions present in a patient whose ulcer is under control.

Some clinics and fasting practitioners do believe in fasting for ulcers. In the first test case of the Master Cleanser (p. 61), Stanley Burroughs claims to have cured a patient with an intractable ulcer. The two main ingredients of the Master Cleanser, citrus and cayenne pepper, are substances that all the physicians had suggested this patient avoid; Dr. Burroughs deduced they might be the only things left to heal the ulcer, and perhaps he is right. The fasting process itself is helpful for ulcers as it reduces stomach acid and aids in tissue healing. Cayenne pepper, although hot, heals mucous membranes and is commonly recommended for ulcers in herbal medicines. So, even though peptic ulcers are on the contraindication list, some people may be helped by fasting, especially with cabbage/vegetable juices.

CONTRAINDICATIONS FOR FASTING		
Underweight	Cardiac arrhythmias	Pre- and postsurgery
Fatigue	Cold weather	Cancer
Low immunity	Pregnancy	Peptic ulcers
Weak heart	Nursing	Nutritional deficiencies
Low blood pressure		Children

As with any therapy, fasting has some potential hazards. Clearly, excessive weight loss and nutritional deficiencies may occur—a response more marked with longer water fasts and less likely with juices as they provide some calories and nutrients. Weakness may occur, or muscle cramps may result from mineral deficits. Sodium, potassium, calcium, magnesium, and phosphorus losses occur initially but diminish after a week. Blood pressure drops, and this can lead to dizziness (especially when changing position from lying to sitting or from sitting to standing). Uric acid levels may rise without adequate fluid intake, although this is rare.

Some research reports that hormone levels change while fasting. Initially, the level of thyroid hormone falls, but it rises again in association with protein-sparing ketosis. Female hormone levels fall, possibly as a result of protein malnutrition, and this can lead to a lessening or loss of menstrual flow. Cessation of periods in women is also seen in longtime vegetarians, particularly those who exercise extensively, arising typically from nutrient depletion. This will usually rebalance with proper diet and nourishment.

Cardiac problems such as arrhythmias can occur with prolonged fasting, especially when there are preexisting problems. Extra beats, both ventricular and atrial, have been seen, and there have even been deaths from serious ventricular arrhythmias (the latter of which occur most often during long water fasts). Similar problems have turned up in people using any nutrient-deficient protein powders, without supervision, as a weight loss tool. All of these risks are minimized with juice fasts of no more than two weeks duration or when basic minerals (potassium, calcium, and magnesium) are supplemented during water fasts. Having our progress monitored through physical exams, blood tests, and even electrocardiograms is another way to protect ourselves from fasting's potential hazards.

Another "side effect" (really a "side benefit") of fasting is the way it affects and changes our personal lives. Often we resist inner guidance, feelings, and desires to do something new or get out of a bad situation, but fasting brings these to the fore. Divorce, job changes, and residential moves are all more likely after fasts, as they stimulate self-realization, enhance our potential, and help us focus on the future. During fasting, many people have new sensitivity and renewed awareness of their job, mate, and home. It does help when couples do programs together. It is good to remember that fasting can be a catalyst for change, and this creates an extra stress during detoxification. However, when we can relax and observe what's going on, it helps to create better understanding. Even though these insights and changes may be traumatic initially, I believe they are ultimately positive and help us follow our true nature.

HOW TO FAST

The general plan for fasting is progressive, usually a moderate approach for new fasters and unhealthy subjects, leading to a stricter program for the more experienced. It is important to build slowly and take time to transition. Although many people do fine even when making extreme changes, such abruptness clearly maximizes the risks of fasting.

A sensible daily plan mixes fasting with eating. Each day can include a twelve- to fourteen-hour period of fasting from early evening through the night, as indeed breakfast was given that name to denote the time where we break the fast of the night. Many people eat very lightly or not at all in the early morning in order to extend their daily fast; this is more important if dinner or snacking extends into the later evening. However, if dinner is at an early time, a good breakfast can be consumed after water intake and some stretching and exercise.

In preparation for our first day of fasting, we may want to take some time (a few days to a week) to eliminate unhealthy foods or habits from our diet. Abstaining from alcohol, nicotine, caffeine, and sugar is very helpful before fasting. Red meats and other animal foods, including milk products and eggs, as well as wheat and baked goods could be avoided for a day or two before fasting, thus easing the transition. *Intake of most nutritional supplements should also be curtailed as these are usually not recommended during a fast.* Many people prepare for their fasts by consuming only fruit and vegetable foods for three or four days. These slowly detoxify the body so that the actual fast will be less intense.

The first one-day fast gives us a chance to see what a short fast can be like. Most of us find that it is not so very difficult and does not cause major distress. Food is abstained from for thirty-six hours, from 8 P.M. one night until 8 A.M. two days later. Most people will feel a little hungry and may experience a few mild symptoms such as a headache or irritability by the end of the fasting day, usually around dinnertime. The first two days are generally challenging for everyone; feeling great usually begins around day three. So take a walk, take a nap, cut your nails, breathe, read a book, pray, and bathe instead of eating.

One of the ironies of fasting is that it can be the most difficult for those who need it the most; in these cases, people must start with the subtle diet changes discussed above. One transition protocol is the one-meal-a-day plan. The meal is usually eaten around 3 P.M.; water, juices, teas, and some fresh fruit or vegetable snacks can be eaten at other times. It is important that the wholesome meal be neither excessive nor rich. Start with a protein and vegetable meal, such as fish and salad or steamed vegetables, or a starch and vegetable meal, such as brown rice and mixed steamed greens, carrots, celery, and zucchini. People on this plan detoxify slowly, lose some weight, and after a few days feel pretty sound. The chance of any strong symptoms developing during this transition time or during a subsequent fast is greatly minimized.

The next goal for those who have done a one-meal-a-day program is a one-day fast. The fasting then progresses to two- and three-day fasts with one or two days between them when light foods and more raw fruits and vegetables are consumed. This allows us to build up to longer lasting five- to ten-day fasts. When the transition is made this slowly, even water fasting can be less intense (although I usually recommend juice fasts).

To avoid being excessively impatient, we need to make and adhere to a plan. It is important to continually observe and listen to your body and even keep notes in a journal. Get to know yourself and your nature. Once we have fasted successfully, we can continue to do one-day fasts weekly or a three-day fast every month if we need them. This experience helps us to reconnect with ourselves and to work toward a goal of optimum health. Meditation, exercise, fresh air and sunshine, massages, and baths are all essential and nourishing during this and any cleansing period.

TIMING OF FASTS

The two key times for natural cleansing are the times of transition into spring and autumn. In Chinese medicine, this transition time between the seasons is about ten days before and after each equinox or solstice. For spring, this period runs from about March 10 through April 1; for autumn, it is from about September 11 through October 2. In cooler climates, where spring weather begins later and autumn weather earlier, the fasting could be scheduled appropriately as it is easier to do when it is warm as the body tends to cool down during fasting.

SPRING MASTER CLEANSER

2 tablespoons freshly squeezed lemon or lime juice
1 tablespoon pure maple syrup (up to 2 tablespoons if you want to drop less weight)
$^1/_{10}$ teaspoon cayenne pepper
8 ounces spring water

Important Notes: Mix and drink 8–12 glasses throughout the day. Eat or drink nothing else except water, laxative herb tea, and peppermint or chamomile tea. Keep the mixture in a glass container (not plastic) or make it fresh each time. Rinse your mouth with water after each glass to prevent the lemon juice from hurting the enamel of your teeth.

For a spring fast, I usually suggest lemon and/or greens as the focus of the cleansing. Diluted lemon water, lemon and honey, or, my favorite, the Master Cleanser can be used.

Fresh fruit or vegetable juices diluted with equal amounts of water will also stimulate cleansing. Some good vegetable choices are carrots, celery, beets, and greens. Soup broths can also be used. Juices with blue-green algae, spirulina, or chlorella provide more energy, as they contain quality protein (amino acids) and are easily assimilated.

Fasting can also be done in other seasons. Summer with the warm weather is a good time to do ten days. Winter cleansing can be one day per month or longer, but warming diets, such as brown rice, vegetables, and miso soup can also be helpful. This can be done for two to three weeks. In autumn, a fast of at least three to five days can

AUTUMN REJUVENATION RATION*

3 cups spring water
1 tablespoon chopped ginger root
1–2 tablespoons miso paste
1–2 stalks green onion, chopped

Chopped cilantro, to taste
1–2 pinches cayenne pepper
2 teaspoons extra virgin olive oil
Juice of $^1/_2$ lemon

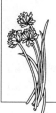

Boil water. Add ginger root. Simmer 10 minutes. Stir in miso paste to taste (do not allow miso paste to boil). Turn off burner. Then add green onion, cilantro, cayenne, olive oil, and lemon juice. Remove from stove and cover to steep for 10 minutes. You may vary ingredient portions to satisfy your palate. Enjoy.
* From Bethany Argisle

be done, using either water or a variety of juices. Juices could include the Master Cleanser, apple and/or freshly made grape juice (usually mixed with a little lemon and water to reduce sweetness), vegetable juices, and warm broths.

How Do We Know How Long to Fast?

We can either follow a specific time schedule or listen closely to our own individual cycles and needs. Paying attention to our energy level, and degree of congestion, and observing our tongue and its coating will offer helpful cleansing guidelines. As we gain some fasting experience, we will become more attuned to specific times when we need to strengthen or lighten our diet and when we need to cleanse. If we are under stress, have been overindulging, or develop some congestive symptoms, we need to lighten our diet and possibly cleanse. The odor of our urine, breath, and sweat are tell-tale signs of cleansing in action.

Breaking a Fast

Ending or stopping a fast and beginning to eat again also takes some monitoring. Things to watch include energy level, weight, detox symptoms, tongue coating, and degree of hunger. If our energy falls for more than a day or if our weight gets too low, we should come off the fast. If symptoms are particularly intense or sudden, it is possible that we need food. Generally, the tongue is a good indicator of our state of toxicity or clarity. With fasting, the tongue usually becomes coated with a white, yellow, or gray film. This signals the body's cleansing process, and it will usually clear when the detox cycle is complete. However, tongue observation is not a foolproof indicator. Some people's tongues are coated very little, while others will remain coated even after cleansing. If in doubt, it is better to make the transition back to food and then cleanse again later. Hunger is another sign of readiness to move back into eating, as it is often minimal during cleansing times. Occasionally, people are very hungry throughout a fast, but most lose interest in food from day three to seven and then experience real, deep-seated hunger once again. This is a sign to eat carefully.

Breaking a fast must be well planned and executed slowly and carefully to prevent the creation of symptoms and sickness. It is suggested that we take half of our total cleansing time to move back into our regular diet, which is hopefully now better planned and more healthful. Our digestion has been at rest, so we need to chew our foods very well. If we have fasted on water alone, we need to prepare our digestive tract with diluted juices, perhaps beginning with a few teaspoons of fresh orange juice in a glass of water and progressing to stronger mixtures throughout the day. Diluted fresh grape or orange juice will stimulate the digestion. Arnold Ehret, a European fasting expert and proponent of the "mucusless" diet, suggests that fruits and fruit juices should not be used right after a meat eater's first fast because they may coagulate intestinal mucus and cause problems. A meat eater's colon bacteria are probably different from a vegetarian's. Consequently, fruit sugars like those in the juices may not be tolerated well; instead, the active gram-positive anaerobic bacteria in the meat eater will produce more toxins. Extra acidophilus supplements continued on a regular basis help shift colon ecology in meat eaters and can even be used during cleanses.

With juice fasting, it is easier to transition back to food. A raw or cooked low-starch vegetable, such as spinach or other greens, is quite appropriate. A little sauerkraut also helps to stimulate the digestive function. A laxative-type meal including grapes, cherries, or soaked or stewed prunes can also be used to initiate eating, as they keep the bowels moving. Some experts say that the bowels should move within an hour or two after the first meal and, if not, an enema should be used. Some people do a saltwater flush before their first day of food by drinking a quart of water containing 2 teaspoons of dissolved sea salt. Be careful. (See more on colon cleansing on page 66.) Our individual transit times vary in response to laxatives and saltwater.

However you make the transition, go slowly, chew well, and do not overeat or mix too many foods at any meal. Start with simple vegetable meals, such as salads or steamed veggies. Fruit should be eaten alone. Soaked prunes or figs are helpful. Well-cooked, watery brown rice or millet is handled well by most people by the second day. From there, progress slowly through grains and vegetables. Some nuts, seeds, or legumes can be added, and then richer protein foods, if these are desired. Returning to food is a crucial time for learning individual responses or reactions. Self-observation gives us an opportunity to see destructive dietary habits and discover specific food intolerances. You may wish to keep notes at this time. If you respond poorly to a food, avoid it for a week or so, and then eat it alone to see how it feels. This is when food allergies may be revealed.

JUICE SPECIFICS

Some juices work better for certain people or conditions. In general, diluted fresh juices of raw organic fruits and vegetables are best. Canned and frozen juices should be avoided. Some bottled juice may be used, but fresh squeezed or extracted is best, as long as it is used soon after processing. Lemon juice, wheat grass, or a little ginger or garlic juice can be added to drinks for vitality and to stimulate cleansing.

Water and other liquids increase waste elimination. Lemon tends to loosen and draw out mucus and is especially useful for liver cleansing. Diluted lemon juice with or without a little honey or the Master Cleanser lemonade loosens mucus quickly, so if this is used we need to cleanse the bowels regularly to prevent getting sick. Most vegetable juices are milder than lemon juice.

Fruit Juices and the Organs or Conditions They Help Heal	Vegetable Juices and the Organs or Conditions They Help Heal
Lemon—liver, gallbladder, allergies, asthma, cardiovascular disease (CVD), colds Citrus—CVD, obesity, hemorrhoids, varicose veins Apple—liver, intestines Pear—gallbladder Grape—colon, anemia Papaya—stomach, indigestion, hemorrhoids, colitis Pineapple—allergies, arthritis, inflammation, edema, hemorrhoids Watermelon—kidneys, edema Black cherry—colon, menstrual problems, gout	Greens—CVD, skin, eczema, digestive problems, obesity, bad breath Spinach—anemia, eczema Parsley—kidneys, edema, arthritis Beet greens—gallbladder, liver, osteoporosis Watercress—anemia, colds Wheat grass—anemia, liver, intestines, bad breath Cabbage—colitis, ulcers Carrots—eyes, arthritis, osteoporosis Beets—blood, liver, menstrual problems, arthritis Celery—kidneys, diabetes, osteoporosis Cucumber—edema, diabetes Jerusalem artichokes—diabetes Garlic—allergies, colds, hypertension, CVD, high fats, diabetes Radish—liver, high fats, obesity Potatoes—intestines, ulcers

Each juice has a certain nutritional composition and probable physiological actions (although these have not been studied extensively). Fresh juices are like natural vitamin pills with a very high assimilation rate that do not require the work of digestion.

The juices of apples, grapes, oranges, and carrots are good cleansing juices but might be minimized for weight loss as they are high in calories. Juices more helpful for weight loss include grapefruit, lemon, cucumber, and greens such as lettuce, spinach, or parsley. Also, a variety of juices can be used in a fast, prepared fresh daily. Keep recipes of your favorite new combinations.

To prepare juices, we want to start with the freshest and most chemical-free fruits and vegetables possible. They should be cleaned or soaked and stored properly. If not organic, they should be peeled, especially if they are waxed. With root vegetables such as carrots or beets, the above-ground ends should be trimmed. Some people drop their vegetables into a pot of boiling water for a minute or so to clean them before juicing. Use organic produce to avoid chemical herbicides and pesticides.

The right juicer is important. The rotary-blade juicers (Champion brand) are very good at squeezing the juice with minimum molecular irritation and are medium in price range. The centrifuge juicers are also fine, but they waste juice left in pulp. The best juicers are the compressors (Norwalk brand), which are more expensive. Blenders are not really juicers (what they produce is more like liquid salad) but can be used to puree soups of make smoothies. These drinks can also be used for a fast since they are high in fiber and nutrients. I once did an energizing week-long fast with two blender drinks a day—fruits in the morning and vegetables in the late afternoon—with teas and water in between.

OTHER ASPECTS OF HEALTHY FASTING

- **Fresh air**—plenty is needed to support cleansing and oxygenation of the cells and tissues.

- **Sunshine**—also needed to revitalize our body; avoid excessive exposure.

- **Water**—bathing is very important to cleanse the skin at least twice daily.

- **Steams and saunas** are also good for providing warmth and supporting detoxification.

- **Skin brushing**—with a dry, soft brush prior to bathing is a good year-round practice as well. This will help clear toxins from the skin.

- **Exercise**—very important to support the cleansing process. It helps to relax the body, clears wastes, and prevents toxicity symptoms. Walking, bicycling, swimming, or other exercise can be done during a fast, although sports that entail risk, danger, or physical contact should be avoided.

- **No drugs**—none should be used during fasts except mandatory prescription drugs. Avoidance of alcohol, nicotine, and caffeine is imperative.

- **Vitamin supplements**—these are not used during fasting, and thus no program of nutrients will follow at the end of this chapter. Supplemental fiber, such as psyllium husks, can help detox the colon. Special chlorophyll foods such as green barley, chlorella, spirulina, or blue-green algae may enhance vitality and purification. Occasionally, some mineral support (especially potassium, calcium, magnesium, with vitamin C) in powdered or liquid forms helps prevent cramps or adds support during an extended fast. Some people even use amino-acid or other vitamin powders. These supplemental nutrients are really best used when consumed with foods. (See Chapter 6 for more on supplements and detoxification.)

- **Colon cleansing**—an essential part of healthy fasting. Some form of bowel stimulation is recommended. Colonic irrigations with water performed by a trained therapist with modern equipment are the most thorough. These can be done at the beginning, midpoint, and end of the fast. It is suggested that enemas be used at least every other day, especially if they are the primary cleansing method. Fasting clinics often suggest that enemas be used daily or several times a day. With these, water alone is used to flush the colon of toxins. It may be helpful for an enema or laxative preparation to be used the day before the fast begins to lessen initial toxicity. Herbal laxatives are commonly taken orally during fasting, and many formulas are available either as capsules or for making tea. These include cascara sagrada, senna leaves, licorice root, buckthorn, rhubarb root, aloe vera, and prepared formulas. The saltwater flush (drinking a quart of warm water with two teaspoons of sea salt dissolved in it) can be used first thing in the morning on alternate days throughout the fast to flush the entire intestinal tract, although it does not work well for everyone. It is not recommended for salt-sensitive or water-retaining people, or for people with hypertension.

- **Work and be creative**—and make plans for your life. Staying busy helps break our ties to food. Most fasters experience greater work energy and more creativity and, naturally, find lots to do.

- **Cleanup**—both our body and our environment: our room, desk, office, closet, and home. If we want to prepare for the new, we need to clear out the old.

- **Joining others in fasting** can generate strong bonds and provide an additional spiritual lift. It creates new supportive relationships and adds levels to existing ones. Most people feel better as their fast progresses—more vital, lighter, less blocked, more flexible, clearer, and more spiritually attuned. For many, it is nice to have someone with whom to share this. Call our clinic or another that offers this service.

- **Avoid the negative influence** of others who may not understand or support us. Remember to listen to your inner guidance and to be aware of any problems. Being in contact with other fasters or sympathetic people who understand benefits of fasting will provide us with the positive, grounded support we need.

- **The economy of fasting** allows us to save time, money, and future health-care costs. Many of us will be inspired to share more of ourselves when we are freed from food.

- **Meditation and relaxation** are other important aspects of fasting that help clear stresses and bring us into contact with ourselves.

- **Spiritual practice and prayer** will affirm our positive attitude and support our meditation and relaxation, providing us with inner fuel to live with purpose and passion.

CONCLUSION

When we overdo it with food or other substances, we need to return to the cycle of a daily night fast of twelve to fourteen hours and eating one main meal and two lighter ones. For low-weight, high-metabolism people, two larger- or three moderately sized meals are probably needed. If we eat a heavier evening meal, we may need only a light breakfast, and vice versa. Through awareness and experience, we can find our individual nutritional needs and fulfill them with ease.

Fasting can easily become both a way of life and an effective dietary practice. Over a period of time we can go from symptom cleansing to preventive fasting. We should support ourselves regularly with a balanced, wholesome diet and fast at specific times to treat symptoms and/or to enhance our vitality and spiritual practice. If we could devote one day per week to purification and a cleansing diet, the path of health would be smooth indeed.

Choosing healthy foods, chewing well, and maintaining good colon function all minimize our need for fasting. However, if we do get out of balance, we can employ one of the oldest treatments known to humans, the instinctive therapy for many illnesses, nature's doctor, therapist, and tool for preventing disease—FASTING!

CHAPTER FOUR

The Detox Diet and Other Purifying Diets

◆

Before we approach the Detox Diet, we first want to give you some preventive medicine guidelines to follow so that you don't need to detoxify as often. Instead, learn to eat and live in a way that creates and supports health, vitality, and longevity. The first step is to follow a nontoxic diet. If we do this regularly, we have less need for cleansing. If we have not been eating this way, we should detoxify first and then make these more permanent changes. And of course, as we exercise and stretch regularly, rest and sleep well, and take a great attitude toward life and others, this all will keep our stress low and our health high.

THE NONTOXIC DIET

- Eat organically grown foods whenever possible.
- Drink filtered (or properly purified) water.
- Eat a natural, seasonal cuisine, focusing on fresh foods as much as possible.
- Include fruits, vegetables, whole grains, legumes, nuts, and seeds, and, for omnivarians, some low- or non-fat dairy products (particularly organic yogurt), fresh fish (not shellfish), and organic poultry.
- Rotate foods, especially common allergens such as milk products, eggs, wheat, and yeast foods.
- Practice food combining, avoiding mixing too many foods per meal and overeating.
- Cook in iron, stainless steel, glass, or porcelain cookware.
- Avoid or minimize red meats, cured meats, organ meats, refined foods, canned foods, sugar, salt, saturated fats, coffee, alcohol, and nicotine.

Another aspect of the nontoxic diet is avoiding drugs (over-the-counter, prescription, and recreational) and substituting natural remedies such as nutritional supplements, herbs, and homeopathic medicines, all of which have fewer side effects.*

Other natural therapies, such as acupuncture, massage, osteopathic, and chiropractic care may help in treating certain problems so that we will not need drugs for them. Avoiding or minimizing exposure to chemicals at home and at work is also important. One way we can do this is by substituting natural cleansers, cosmetics, and clothing.

THE DETOX DIET

One of my favorite cleansing/detox programs is the Detox Diet. It is a simple eating program that I have used with many thousands of people. I find it to be a great catalyst for healing, providing more energy, fewer debilitating symptoms (such as aches and pains or congestion and allergies), and the inspiration necessary for making permanent changes in diet and lifestyle habits.

When I did my first 3-week Detox Diet, I learned to chew my food thoroughly for the first time in my life. I felt more nourished on less food and I experienced less bloating, gas, and fullness in the several hours after eating. My weight dropped five pounds per week and I felt clearer, more energized, and less congested.

Over the last ten years, I have prescribed this Detox Diet (as a healing diet and catalyst for habit changes) for those with obvious congestion-toxicity concerns, such as people with high blood pressure who are also overweight and stressed, those with arthritis and joint pains, allergies, or recurrent sinus problems, or those with back pains or lymphatic congestion. Most people experience similar results—a couple of days of transition with occasional fatigue, irritability, hunger, or increased congestion. Usually by the third day they start to feel cleaner, clearer, lighter, stronger, and more present in their body, aware of the way it responds to food and liquid intake. Their symptoms of congestion and pain diminish and even disappear. It is very gratifying for them and me and often represents a long-term change, and it certainly makes my job more enjoyable and rewarding.

---

* See p. 178 for advice on transitioning from pharmaceutical to natural therapies.

Other Diets for Detoxification

The following detoxifying and purifying diet programs cover a wide range of caloric needs to help you tailor a program that's just right for you. They include the Original Detox Diet, the Smoothie Cleanse, and the Juice Cleanse. These varying programs allow some diversity to help guide you through the most appropriate cleanse depending on your body type and needs, the time of year, the length of time you would like to cleanse, and your individual food sensitivities and caloric needs. The next chapter, Transitional Diets, will help you to move out of the Detox Diet or Cleansing Program and create a healthy, long-term diet. The specific Life-Long Detox Diet, including a Hypoallergenic Plan with avoidance of regular use of SNACCs (Sugar, Nicotine, Alcohol, Caffeine, and Chemicals), will be discussed with a reference to the seasonal menu plan and healthy eating that is reviewed thoroughly in the companion to this book, *A Cookbook for All Seasons*. Incorporating the concepts of the nontoxic diet previously listed also offer the keys for any good diet.

Deciding What to Do with a Practitioner's Help

Working with a practioner's guidance for detoxification can be helpful. When I set up an initial personalized detox/cleansing program, I evaluate each individual with a health history, physical exam, biochemical tests, dietary review, and other relevant tests based on the person's needs. These tests could include digestive analyses for function as well as microbes (both normal and abnormal), blood mineral levels, and an evaluation of food reactions through blood. By interpreting the patient's current symptoms and disease as a result of his/her diet, lifestyle, and genetic patterns, and by then considering his/her current health goals, we can create a plan together. As is true with any healing process, the plan must be reevaluated and fine-tuned to the individual to make it work optimally over time.

If the patient is deficient in nutrients and/or energy, she may need a higher-protein, higher-nutrient rebuilding diet—greater nourishment rather than a cleansing program to improve her health. Fatigue, mineral deficiencies, and low organ functions may call for this more supportive, nourishing diet, and not so much detoxifying. However, even in these circumstances, short three-day cleanses or avoiding foods like wheat, sugar, and milk products, can help eliminate old debris and prepare the body to build with healthier blocks.

Our individual detox (purifying) programs do change, as our needs often vary with time. For instance, my own personal program has changed in intensity over the decades. Initially, fasts were very powerful, transformative, and healing for me. Now I feel much cleaner most of the time, and I usually notice less effect from a fast. If I do get congested with different foods, travel, or when under stress, a few days of juices or light eating will make a big difference. I ate a low-protein, high-complex-carbohydrate vegetarian diet for a number of years; now my mild detox consists of more strengthening protein-vegetable meals. Fresh fish with lots of vegetables satisfies and energizes me more now than it did in the past. My previous higher-starch diet led me to overeat in order to feel nourished. This new diet has let me reduce calories and weight while feeling stronger and healthier. And this too, I am sure, will change over time.

How to Decide What to Do

Here's a few other tips on how to choose which cleanse or detox program to do, how long to go, and how to move from one to the other. The best way to think about them is to see the Detox Diet as the basic plan, moving along to more intensity with the Smoothie Cleanse, and last, the most extreme, the Juice Cleanse. In actuality, water fasting is the most intense, but we do not recommend that here, as it should be done under supervision in most situations. In our groups, we often use these different levels of the detox programs as stepping stones toward our longer range goal of cleaning up our bodies, losing weight, clearing symptoms, and creating overall healing. Everyone feels lighter and clearer with the feeling of making a fresh start. **The transition back into the right diet for each of you is the most important part of the whole process.** If you just go back to your old diet (unless it is already very good), it likely isn't worth the whole effort, since your body and health will soon return to a lesser level as well. **The key idea for this detoxification process is to come out the other side with more awareness and healthier habits, and then a healthier body.** Each of these following programs can be done exclusively as well, such as the Detox Diet for two to three weeks, the Smoothie Cleanse for one to two weeks, or the Juice Cleanse for three to ten or more days, all depending on the body state and needs.

A good example of a two to three week process can start with the Detox Diet for about a week, then shift over to Smoothies and Juices, either combined together over the day or done exclusively. Many people can combine the liquid cleansing with the Detox Diet, where they do juices through the day, but have a salad or steamed veggies at lunch and/or dinner. You will be learning, or really re-learning, to listen to their bodies and adapt as they are instinctually guided. And in actuality, that is a common and extremely empowering process for most participants in my groups. From the cleansing week, you can move back into the Detox Diet for another week. Make sure you are balancing with some supplements (see Chapter 6), drinking water, and doing your exercise. And then, you can move into the Transition Diets in Chapter 6, and hopefully not through into the bread and cheese, or candy and soda plan. Stay with it as the habits can change just by making the good choices and eating the good foods. Think about what you can eat, what's right for you, and not what you can't have. Your bowl is not half empty, but half full on the way to flowing over the brim with great health. Good luck and good health!

The Detox Diet & Daily Menu Plan

This is based on *The Detox Diet,* a book that was first published in late 1996. Many thousands of people have successfully cleansed with this simple menu plan. This program can be followed for just one day or up to three to four weeks. The diet includes wholesome foods such as whole grains, vegetables, fruits, and teas. It can also be expanded to include dressings, dips and sauces as well as drinks to help those who would like to follow the diet longer. The Smoothie Cleanse will provide added nutritional drinks for those who need more calories and/or protein for energy, weight maintenance, and muscle support. Even adding smoothies to the Detox Diet makes the overall program more caloric and nutritional, and thus prevents weight loss. However, it also may be less detoxifying. When following a longer-term program, we also suggest adding fish (or other good proteins) to the program if you are active, have hypoglycemia, or just generally need more protein and calories. The added protein helps to make this a more balanced diet over time, as the more stringent plan is not

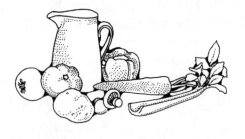

THE NEW DETOX DIET DAILY MENU PLAN

Upon rising:
Two glasses of water (filtered), one glass with half a lemon squeezed into it.

Breakfast:
One piece of fresh fruit (at room temperature), such as an apple, pear, banana, a citrus fruit, or some grapes. Chew well, mixing each bite with saliva.

Fifteen to thirty minutes later: One bowl of cooked whole grains—millet, brown rice, amaranth, or quinoa are the best choices. Oatmeal may be used since this tends to be many folks' favorite as a breakfast grain, but it does contain some glueten.

For flavoring, use 2 tablespoons of fruit juice for sweetness or 1 tablespoon Better Butter with a little sea salt or tamari for a more savory taste.

Lunch:
(Noon–1 P.M.) One to two medium bowls of steamed vegetables. Use a variety, including roots, stems, and greens. For example, potatoes or yams, green beans, broccoli or cauliflower, carrots or beets, asparagus, kale or chard, and cabbage. One to two teaspoons of dressing, such as Better Butter, can be used. Be sure to chew well!

Dinner:
(5–6 P.M.) Same as lunch. For any who are fatigued, or feel they just need protein, 3 to 4 ounces of fish, poultry, or bean, can be added at this meal or better even at 3 to 4 P.M. See about quality animal proteins on page 87.

Special drinks: (11 A.M. and 3 P.M.)
This is the water that is collected from steaming the vegetables. It contains many nutrients and offers a more alkaline balance for the body. A bit of veggie salt or garlic salt can be used.

Before retiring:
Consume no additional foods after dinner. Drink only water and herbal teas.

Note: The times of eating are relatively important, especially finishing eating by 6 P.M. or so, or by nightfall at the latest if your schedule can't conform. Having that rest from food overnight is important to the detox process.

Better Butter Recipe

Makes 32 servings (can make half this amount by halving recipe)

Better Butter spreads easily and is lower in cholesterol and saturated fat than butter alone. Flaxseed or canola oil can also be used.

1 cup extra virgin olive oil (organic if possible)

1 cup (or 2 sticks) of organic butter, at room temperature

In a glass bowl, combine the olive oil and butter until well mixed. Cover and store in the refrigerator for up to 2 weeks.

completely balanced. Adding some of the blue-green algaes does add some amino acids and protein.

SEASONAL VEGETABLE SUGGESTIONS

Try steaming basic combinations that include some root vegetables, tubers, stems, leafy greens, and vegetable "fruits" (from flowering vines that give such veggies as zucchini, green beans, and peppers).

~ SPRING ~

Asparagus, baby carrots, spring garlic, red chard, beets, leeks, broccoli, sugar peas.
Wild greens such as mustard, sorrel, or collard, and steamed artichoke.

~ SUMMER ~

Zucchini, new potatoes, green beans, carrots, onion.
Beets and beet greens, yellow squash, bell pepper, and eggplant.

~ AUTUMN ~

Broccoli, cabbage, potato, pumpkin, celery, spinach.
Cauliflower, onion, zucchini, carrots, chard, and string beans.

~ WINTER ~

Broccoli, cabbage, potato, kale, spinach, chard.
Butternut squash, onion, cauliflower, collard greens, and Jerusalem artichoke.

To season, add a little bit of sea salt, vegetable salt, fresh garlic or dried garlic without additives, or cayenne for warmth. Better Butter is a must for this Detox Diet as it prevents deficiencies of essential fatty acids. The mixture of butter and extra virgin olive oil provides fatty acids to nourish and support the tissues.

SMOOTHIE CLEANSE

The Smoothie Cleanse is a general short-term (1 to 2 weeks) diet of fruit smoothies and vegetable juices and smoothies, which can be supplemented with green products for energy and with protein powder for those who have a higher caloric or protein need. Adding protein powder to your smoothies is especially important for those who do not want to lose weight, for athletes who don't wish to lower muscle mass, and for those with hypoglycemia (low blood sugar issues). Good quality protein powders are available from rice, milk (whey proteins), or soy (organic soy only).

Smoothies are easy to make, delicious, and only require minimal equipment and preparation. All you need is a blender (unless you wish to squeeze or press your own juices first, which is the ideal). You can personalize your smoothie to include your favorite flavors, the protein you need for an active lifestyle, as well as hide potent detoxifiers in those cool, rich drinks.

The basic formula for a smoothie is 1 cup (per person) of liquid such as fruit juice, rice milk, almond milk, organic soymilk, oat milk, or multi-grain milk. (Note: We are having you avoid cow's milk for a variety of health-related reasons, yet, some people still favor cow's milk and whey protein powder, or goat's milk and its products.) Add 1 cup of fruit, either fresh or frozen, and you have your base drink. Smoothies are so rich and creamy (a half to one banana helps with this quality) that you can hide ingredients such as ground flaxseed, wheat germ, flaxseed oil, and protein powders without changing the flavor too much. On top of that you can add nutrients such as probiotics (healthy bacteria such as acidophilus), algae, vitamin C, and many other supplements. This is a great benefit to those on the run and for those who have a hard time swallowing supplements.

Drink your smoothies as soon as possible after making them so the ingredients are fresh and have not oxidized.

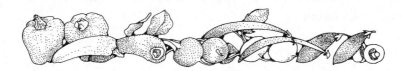

THE SMOOTHIE CLEANSE DAILY MENU PLAN

Upon Rising:

Two glasses of water (filtered), one glass with half a lemon squeezed into it.

Breakfast:

One piece of fresh fruit (at room temperature), such as an apple, pear, banana, a citrus fruit, or some grapes. Chew well, mixing each bite with saliva. This awakens your digestion.

Fifteen to thirty minutes later: A smoothie made with fruit and juice or milk alternative. Add ingredients to meet your specific needs, such as protein powder if you are active. Remember to chew your smoothie to mix your saliva with the rich fluid, which helps begin the digestive process.

Lunch:

(Noon–1 P.M.) A smoothie or a fresh vegetable juice.

Snack:

(3 P.M.) A smoothie or a fresh vegetable juice.

Dinner:

(5–6 P.M.) A smoothie or a fresh vegetable juice.

Before retiring:

Consume no additional foods after dinner. Drink only water and herbal teas.

Smoothie Example Recipes

See Chapter 13 for more smoothie recipes

High Energy Banana Shake

Serves 1

Bananas provide electrolytes and easily absorbed calories to boost energy.

1 cup milk or milk alternative (rice, almond, oat, or soy)
1 banana (fresh or frozen)
1–2 tablespoons protein powder

Blend all ingredients in a food processor or blender until smooth and drink immediately.

Berry Cooler

Serves 1

Berries contain cleansing fiber and antioxidants. Frozen berries create more of a milkshake effect than fresh. Protein powder can be added to this or any smoothie for those who have higher caloric needs.

1 cup milk, milk alternative, or juice
½–1 cup berries (fresh or frozen)
1–2 tablespoons protein powder (optional)
1 banana (optional)

Blend all ingredients in a food processor or blender until smooth and drink immediately.

Carrot Smoothie

Serves 1

Carrots contain powerful antioxidants and although they cannot be juiced in a blender, carrot juice can be added to any smoothie as a base ingredient. Freshly made carrot juice from your home juicer is best or from the local natural food store (many make fresh juice), or buy freshly bottled juices. If you use bottled vegetable juices, make sure you get them without added sodium.

1 cup carrot juice (fresh or bottled)
2 tablespoons apple juice
1 tablespoon fresh lemon juice
Ice (optional)

Blend all ingredients in a food processor or blender until smooth and drink immediately.

THE JUICE CLEANSE DIET

This three- to ten-day deeper cleanse is the perfect spring cleanse. The popular Master Cleanser (see Chapter 3) is an integral part of the program, which also may include vegetable juices, fruit juices, and vegetables broths.

The juice cleanse diet is a short-term, effective purifying program consisting of nutrient-rich vegetable and fruit juices. Those who want to lose weight, increase the rate of toxin clearing, and have lower caloric needs because they are not extremely active are all candidates for this diet. Regular exercise is still suggested to burn calories and get or stay in shape.

If you haven't experienced fresh juices before, you are in for a big surprise. They are so packed with nutrients that they are very energizing. Fruits and vegetables contain easily absorbed vitamins and minerals, calories for immediate energy production, and vital phytonutrients. These naturally occurring plant nutrients protect us from disease, help heal imbalances, and accelerate the healing process.

To make fresh juices, which are superior to bottled juices, you will need a juicer. The centrifugal force juicers are easy to clean and extract juice well from the pulp of the plants. If you have an orange juice squeezer, you can make fresh citrus juice. However, investing in a juicer will give you the ability to make your own fresh vegetable juices, which are the most vitally alive.

Juices are usually a concoction of various fruits or vegetables. For example, apples with lemon and ginger are warming and enhance digestion, while a combination of carrots, celery, and lemon is refreshing and energizing.

It's important to drink freshly made juices as soon as possible (ideally immediately) so that the nutrients are not exposed to air and light for very long. Some of the vitamins and phytonutrients can oxidize and be lost over time, ranging from minutes to days.

To vary and simplify the juice cleanse or if you are wishing to do it longer, some other detoxifying foods can be eaten if just drinking liquids is too challenging or you are needing to add more fruit and calories. Vegetable soups can be consumed, as can eating fresh fruits and vegetables such as celery, carrots, jicama, apples, pears, oranges, and so forth. See Chapter 13 for recipes and Chapter 3 for more juice ideas. Use in-season and organic fruits and vegetables as much as possible. (See the Seasonal Vegetable suggestions list on page 74 as well.)

THE JUICE CLEANSE DAILY MENU PLAN

Upon Rising:
Two glasses of water (filtered), one glass with half a lemon squeezed into it.

Breakfast:
3–4 eight-ounce glasses of Master Cleanser (consumed over the morning) or one piece of fresh fruit (at room temperature), such as an apple, pear, a citrus fruit, or some grapes. Chew well, mixing each bite with saliva. This awakens your digestion.

Morning:
Several 6–8 ounce glasses of fresh fruit or vegetable juices. (In place of or after master cleanser.) These can be diluted with water, up to half. Apples, grapes, and some lemon make a great fruit juice mix. Fresh grapes and freshly made organic grape juice are also favorites and a healing cleanse program.

Lunch:
(Noon–1 P.M.) A 12-ounce glass of fresh vegetable, Master Cleanser, or fruit juice.

Snack:
(3 P.M.) 6–12 ounces of fresh vegetable juice.

Carrot, beet, and celery are great together. Some greens, such as spinach can be added, or some people like an occasional shot of wheatgrass juice. Some ginger, garlic, and/or lemon can be added to the veggie juice.

Dinner:
(5–6 P.M.) A 12-ounce glass of fresh vegetable juice or some vegetable broth, made from fresh vegetables.

Special Drinks:
(11 A.M. and 3 P.M.) Herbal teas or sparkling water.

Before retiring:
Consume no additional foods after dinner. Drink only water and herbal teas.

Juice Example Recipes

See Chapter 13 for more juice recipes

To make the following recipes you will need a home juicer.

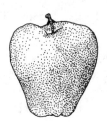

Apple Breeze

Serves 1

This refreshing juice is fairly low in calories and rich in nutrients. This is the perfect drink after a steam, yoga, or stretching session.

2 apples, seeded
2 stalks celery
¼ lemon

Juice according to your machine's instructions and serve immediately. Serve over ice or with a mint leaf or lemon wedge for a festive addition.

Lemon Veggie Delight

Serves 1

This light vegetable juice has a sweet edge from the carrots and a bit of zip from the lemon. You can add any greens you happen to have on hand as most greens such as bok choy (Chinese cabbage), spinach, and garden greens all taste wonderful with carrot and lemon.

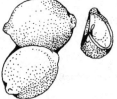

4 carrots
2 stalks celery
4 kale leaves
1 lemon

Juice according to your machine's instructions and drink immediately.

Fresh Tomato Juice

Serves 1

Use the ripest tomatoes possible. Garden tomatoes are exquisite juiced fresh.

2 medium tomatoes
½ red bell pepper
Optional: celery, carrots, yellow or orange bell peppers, a small amount of onion or 1–2 cloves of garlic for a zesty finish.

Juice according to your machine's instructions and drink immediately.

Sweet Beet Elixir

Serves 1

Beet roots have been used in many cultures as a detoxifying juice. Beets are rich in potassium, folic acid, glutathione, and phytoesterols.

1 to 2 beets (with greens if desired)
2 stalks celery
1 to 2 carrots
2 kale leaves
Optional: more carrot if you like, beet greens, or a wedge of lemon.

Juice ingredients together.

Apple Tonic

Serves 1

The pie spice addition to the juice turns it into a comfort drink. Also apple juice is a natural, gentle laxative that is soothing to the digestive tract.

2 apples, seeded
6 ounces boiling water
Large pinch of apple pie spice

Juice according to your machine's instructions. Pour juice into a large mug, add boiling water and stir in the spice mix. Drink immediately.

Note: Because juice fasting is such a powerful detoxifier, it frequently causes temporary detox symptoms, such as headaches, fatigue, irritability, bad breath, skin odor, skin eruptions, and a white coating on the tongue. These symptoms, which are a sure sign that your metabolism is healing, pass in a couple of days, and are generally replaced with a very pleasant sense of calmness, great energy, and a feeling of satisfaction. Detox symptoms, however, can also occur with other types of elimination diets.

THE LIFELONG DETOX DIET

This is similar to the nontoxic diet. Avoid SNACCs and common reactive foods, such as wheat and cow's milk products, or at most rotate them into your diet every few days. Many people have problems with wheat and dairy products, and sugar. However, to consume a diet in these modern times that is void of bread, cheese, or an occasional sweet treat is rather extreme. Just consider them as treats.

That being said, many of these foods are habits and comfort foods, and once we clear them and see that we feel better, have more energy, and stay trimmer, we just find that it's not that difficult to avoid them and eat healthier foods.

The next chapter gives you a more complete picture of moving back into your health-generating diet. There are options in the Transitional Diets chapter and in *A Cookbook for All Seasons*, there is a healthy, clean, balanced, and natural diet for life.

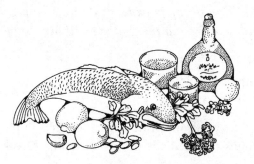

CHAPTER FIVE

Transitional Diets: Moving Forward to Your New Healthy Diet

TRANSITIONING TO YOUR NEW DAILY DIET

When you are making the transition back to your daily diet you may be making more changes to create a satisfying diet replete with comfort foods and occasional treats without reintroducing too many toxins. This can be a simple and fun process with a little guidance and a few tips. Transitioning from each of the specific detox cleanses or diets has its own considerations. The following tips should help you add foods back into your diet through the transition phase.

Detox Diet—With this diet you have already been eating some whole grains and vegetables and now you can expand to include a wider variety of whole grains such as millet, quinoa, and brown rice. Also you can now increase protein and good oil foods such as fish, nuts and seeds, beans, and healthy oils such as flaxseed oil and extra virgin olive oil. See the menu plan on page 73.

Smoothie Cleanse—Start by adding protein powder to your smoothies if you haven't already. Rice protein is a good choice, with other options being soy (organic and non-GMO whenever possible), or even whey (milk extract) powder, which tends to be better tolerated than milk. Nut butters can also be added to smoothies to increase the protein content. Then add more fruits and raw or steamed vegetables into your meal plan. Over several days of the Smoothie Cleanse, you can begin adding whole grains, beans, fish, some nuts and seeds, and healthy oils back into your diet.

The Juice Cleanse Program—Transition slowly by adding pureed fruit (or chew very thoroughly) such as applesauce, berry puree, and fruit smoothies into your plan. During this phase you can also start eating a variety of steamed vegetables, especially steamed greens, plus some light salads with olive oil and lemon or balsamic vinegar.

Again, remember to chew well. Start by adding small amounts of protein (protein powder) to the smoothies; this gets your digestive tract prepared for heavier foods. Do this for at least two days, and then you can begin to eat cooked whole grains, fish, beans, seeds, and oils again. Sprouted beans and seeds are also great.

Many people who follow a detox diet will find that allergic symptoms disappear during their program. This may be because a food that was causing some reaction was removed from the diet. The most common allergens are what I call "The Sensitive Seven" (from my book, *The False Fat Diet*): wheat, cow's milk, sugar, corn, soy, eggs, peanuts, and, of course, all the products made from these foods. Wait to reintroduce these items into your diet until you have first added back in vegetables, fruits, fish, legumes (except soy and peanuts), whole grains, and some nuts and seeds, such as almonds, filberts, and sunflower seeds. At a later time, you can add the Sensitive Seven foods back into the diet, one at a time, and watch for any reaction. This way you'll be able to identify any food reactions. This is true even for other common foods like almonds or potatoes. Awareness of your body and any reactions to a food or meal is a valuable process for what you have invested your time and energy into already.

Choose one of these common sensitive foods to add back into your diet. Eat small amounts at first and then work up over the coming days to eating more of that particular food. If you still feel fine, you are probably not reacting to that food. Then you can try adding the next food back into your diet and so on. Because of many factors, reactions may not be clear and you still may have questions. Typically, when you have avoided a reactive food, you will show a more significant and clear reaction when you bring it back into your diet. However, sometimes if you are mildly reactive, it may take a few exposures to notice any reactions to the accumulative effect. You may feel more tired, have an upset digestion (common with wheat reintroduction), nasal congestion, or a return of other allergy symptoms.

With the most congesting foods, like meats and dairy products, try only small amounts at first (including goat milk and cheeses). If you feel tired, have digestive upset, sinus stuffiness, or other areas of mucus production then you may be reacting to that food. If these reactions occur, you should avoid particular reactive foods for at least a couple of weeks before re-challenging yourself again. If it's difficult to figure out what you are reacting to, you may want to get a food allergy blood test to help you identify what foods are triggering your reactions. These tests vary in their accuracy (or more, their clinical relevance), yet they can be quite helpful in some people. You can read more about this process and these tests in my book, *The False Fat Diet*.

Adding Protein Back into Your Diet

Slowly reintroduce protein into your diet. It can take several days for your body to get used to more protein and other heavier foods coming in, especially after a juice or smoothie cleanse. Your digestive tract will need to respond to the protein foods such as beans, peas, and lentils, and even more with meats and dairy foods by secreting additional hydrochloric acid and digestive enzymes specific to proteins. For example, if you ate a big bowl of chili or a large serving of meat right after a cleansing diet, you may not be able to digest it well, which generally results in gas and constipation, and a very heavy feeling in your body. Some people have a harder time digesting animal foods that have a higher fat content, which include red meats, poultry, fish, cheese, or eggs. In this case, supplementing with hydrochloric acids (HCl as betaine hydro-chloride, often with pepsin, a protein digestant) and/or digestive enzymes may be necessary. Digestive enzymes help break down the carbohydrates, fats, and protein in your diet while HCl helps break down fat and protein. Enzyme supplements and HCl are available from natural food markets, or these supplements may be prescribed by nutritionists and nutritional doctors.

Eating Grains Again

Whole grains such as amaranth, oats, millet, quinoa, and brown rice are complex carbohydrates rich in nutrients and fiber. Start with just one serving a day and slowly add whole grains back into your diet, up to three or four servings. If you tend to be a carbohydrate overeater and are watching your weight, you may wish to limit your grains and go even more slowly in bringing them back into your regular diet. Overall, grains are healthy, high-fiber, foods with decent nutritional value, and this supports good elimination. On the other hand, as stated, you may want to limit your dietary grains; some people do best without any in their diet.

However, if you need to maintain or gain weight, you may want to eat more grains, as well as nuts and seeds. In general, we suggest most people limit their bread and baked good (all made from grains) intake, because there are many healthier choices in the food chain. We suggest you avoid wheat products as long as you can. Yet, good whole-grain dishes are an important part of a healthier, balanced, and more vegetarian, Earth-based diet. See Chapter 13 for a few simple and delicious whole-grain recipes.

Beans, Peas, Lentils, Nuts, and Seeds

Legumes are nutritious partly because they contain so much fiber (plus protein and complex carbohydrate), which helps to release calories into your blood stream slowly, allowing time to burn those calories as energy and thus avoiding fat storage. But all that fiber is hard for some people to digest and you may want to take digestive enzymes for the first week or two that you are eating those foods again. Also many beans, lentils, nuts, and seeds can be sprouted in your own kitchen. Sprouting them makes them much easier to digest and more nourishing. There are also sprouted grain and bean products available in natural food stores.

How to Continue Avoiding SNACCS

Now that you have weaned yourself off of the SNACCs (Sugar, Nicotine, Alcohol, Caffeine, and Chemicals), you'll want to protect yourself from them as you transition back into your daily diet. However, certain challenges may arise as you face old routines that once included these substances.

Ideally you will find alternatives to replace them if that is needed. But if you choose to have a cup of coffee or an occasional drink, you can rotate them in and partake in each as a special treat rather than a daily addictive habit, and then you can still maintain your good health. Your body will be able to detoxify these chemicals given the breaks from them. Remember, it's the daily and long-term use and abuse of these substances/drugs that lead to most of their deleterious effects, much as unhealthy aspects of our diets, such as high-fat, high calories, and low fiber take decades to cause increases in cancer and cardiovascular problems.

Let's just look at sugar as an example. Now that you have been avoiding it, your taste buds may be more sensitive to sweet foods. You may find that candies and sugar laden foods taste awfully sweet and you may no longer have a taste for them at all; you likewise may appreciate the natural sweetness more of an apple, some cherries, or a carrot. If you do choose to indulge in something a little sweet you can choose from healthier options. See example recipes in Chapter 13.

For those who do decide to enjoy an occasional cigarette, be sure your tobacco is high quality, organic, and free of chemicals. The manufacturers of most tobacco products use hundreds of chemicals in the processing of the tobacco, many of which are harmful and toxic. Also, the papers that wrap the tobacco into a cigarette are treated

QUALITY ANIMAL FOODS

Poultry—Avoid mass-market, feed-lot chicken and turkey because many of the big companies raise their chickens in inhumane ways, which stresses the animals, so they get sick more often and are given more antibiotics. Also, they may be given growth hormones and are fed low quality foods, like genetically engineered soybean feed and animal parts. The better choice is "free range" birds (meaning they are not "couped" up) that are veggie fed, meaning they are fed only plant products. Also wild game is exceptionally healthy as they have a higher level of essential fatty acids due to their natural diet of fruits, seeds, berries, and insects.

Beef and Beef Products—The very best beef is from cows that were not sent to a feed lot. Look for the term "grass-fed," which indicates the animal was only fed grass and natural range plants rather than corn or fattening grains on a feed lot. When the animals are fattened to increase their value, the fat composition of the meat changes drastically. The saturated fat and cholesterol levels go up and the healthy essential fatty acid levels come down. Also look for "no hormones," "no antibiotics," and "organic."

Dairy Products—Organic dairy products are the highest quality and now widely available in the United States and Canada. The term *organic* means that the product is free of Bovine Growth Hormone and antibiotics, and the animal was fed an organic, vegetarian diet. Look for "No BGH," "Non-GMO" (Genetically Modified Organism), or "Organic" on milk, cheese, sour cream, yogurt, kefir, and butter. Reason: Many of the most toxic chemicals are stored in the fats of the animals, and since most dairy products have fats, these chemicals pass to us too easily. The cleaner the better is helpful in this area.

Eggs—Look for "free-range" chicken eggs, which indicates the hens were able to run around in fresh air. Also "organic eggs" means the hens were fed only organic feed. Also you can go one step further and get eggs that say "Omega-3 Fatty Acids," and this tells you that the chickens were fed flaxseed. The hens convert the flaxseed into essential fatty acids that ends up in the eggs, making them even more nutritious.

Fish—Generally eating smaller fish is better these days as they are younger and have had less time to accumulate toxins. Also, eating wild fish is usually much healthier over farmed fish as wild fish have eaten natural foods and are rich in essential fatty acids, while farmed fish are typically low in those beneficial oils. Farmed fish are often fed genetically engineered soybean feed, which is higher in herbicides and other chemical residues. And if that's not enough reason to avoid farmed fish, you should be aware that the fish may be injected with Red Dye #40 if the flesh is too pale to sell at the market. So choose wild salmon or small fish such as sardines, anchovies, shad, herring, snapper, and so forth. When you have a choice, choose the smaller varieties of fish. For example, tuna in the can is generally yellow fin, which is fairly large, but albacore tuna is a smaller fish, and thus the better choice between the two.

with chemicals that are known toxins. One company that offers nontoxic tobacco is American Spirit Organic Tobacco and another called Rizla makes chemical-free paper (www.rizla.com).

To completely avoid chemicals you'll want to stay away from processed meats such as lunch meats, salami, bologna, hot dogs, bacon, and some other deli meats. Be sure to read the label on the meats to see if they contain MSG, nitrates, preservatives, sugar, and food coloring, most of which you want to avoid in any regularity. Choose healthier alternatives such as veggie dogs, a beef-like product made of soy. In fact, just about every meat product is now available in a soy form, including salami, Canadian bacon, and so forth.

There are also many options and substitutes for cow's milk products, including rice, almonds, and soy bases used to make milks, cheeses, and ice creams. If you do want cow's milk and other animal products, choose higher quality animal products such as organic milk and cheeses, grass-fed beef, free-range chicken (no antibiotics, and some are even organic in that they are fed only organic foods), lean beef products, and small wild fish (instead of farm-raised fish). This is an important topic in these modern days, so let's look at it a little deeper.

From Simple to Complex Carbohydrates

Refined flour breaks down in our digestive tracts into sugar within minutes and more quickly than whole-grain products. So if you really want to avoid sugar, you'll want to limit the simple carbohydrates found in refined flour products including white bread, pasta, bagels, pretzels, many cereals, plus crackers, donuts, cakes, pies, and so forth. If you read the labels, most of these products also have added sugars. It's easy to find healthier whole-wheat and whole-grain alternatives of most baked goods these days, yet a little more difficult to find baked goods with low sugars. You'll need to read food labels to find the healthiest products.

Avoid hydrogenated oil products including margarines, most packaged baked goods, most crackers and cookies, and fried foods, especially commercial potato and corn chips, which contain partially hydrogenated vegetable oils. As with baked goods, there are healthier versions of chips using organic ingredients, olive oil, and even baked chips that are not fried.

Sugar Alternatives

Sugar is one of the most commonly addictive substances in North America (and the world) and one of the most damaging. The other extreme is synthetic sweeteners such as aspartame and saccharin. Synthetic sweeteners are made in laboratories by chemical companies such as Monsanto and have been linked to brain tumors and bladder cancer. The CDC (Centers for Disease Control) gets more complaints about people who have had headaches and joint pain from these chemical sweeteners than any other food products. We recommend that you avoid these toxins.

However, there are delicious alternatives to sugar, such as barley malt syrup, brown rice syrup, and stevia, a naturally sweet herbal leaf that is available in powders and liquids. Also you can replace sugar in baking with puréed dates or prunes, which make chewy moist cookies or applesauce, and which replaces the sugar and the fat in a recipe. There are many wonderful baking books to help guide you. (See recommended reading list page 240.) See additional recipes for healthier baked goods in Chapter 13. Here's one example for you.

Almond Power Cookies

Makes 20 servings

1 cup barley flour or oat flour
1½ cups oat flakes or oatmeal
1 teaspoon baking soda or 2 egg whites
½ teaspoon salt
2 teaspoons ground cinnamon
¼ cup extra virgin olive oil

½ cup brown rice syrup
1 teaspoon almond extract
2 teaspoons vanilla extract
½ cup almond butter
1 banana, mashed (pureed prunes or raisins may be substituted)

Note: If you don't have almond butter try peanut butter, hazelnut butter, or cashew butter instead.

Preheat oven to 350°F. In a medium bowl, combine flour, oat flakes, baking soda, salt, and cinnamon. Mix well.

In a large bowl, combine the remaining ingredients and mix thoroughly. Add the flour mixture to the oil mixture and combine thoroughly. Onto a nonstick baking sheet, drop the dough in 2-tablespoon-sized balls and bake for 10 minutes.

GENERAL RECOMMENDATIONS FOR A HEALTHY DIET

5–10 servings of vegetables per day

3–4 servings of fruit per day

4–6 or more servings of whole grains

6–8 (8 ounce) glasses of purified water

2–4 servings of a variety of protein foods daily. Include:
      1–2 servings of legumes (beans, peas, lentils) daily
      3–4 servings of fish per week
      1 handful of nuts or seeds per day

What to Eat to Stay Healthy

Eat foods that are in their whole form, as unprocessed as possible, just as Nature made them. (As I state in my book, *Staying Healthy with the Seasons,* eat as close to Nature as possible. Every step away from the whole food is a drop in vitality and nourishment.) Choose brown rice instead of white rice, steel-cut oats rather than minute oatmeal, whole fruit rather than fruit juice, and so forth. Buy or grow the purest food possible. Shop your farmer's market if that's available. Use organic produce, grains, and animal products, especially butter, whenever you can. Try to eat at least *five to seven servings of fresh vegetables and fruits every day.* The focus of a healthy diet is fresh vegetables and adding other whole foods to balance that. Search out the highest quality fish in your area. Avoid the large fishes (examples: swordfish, tuna, and shark), which may contain more ocean toxins, such as mercury, and avoid farmed fish, which test higher for mercury and other chemicals. Instead eat albacore tuna, wild salmon, and small fish, such as sardines.

Daily Oil

Extra virgin olive oil is our favorite oil for cooking and salad dressings. It is a clean choice. "Extra virgin" means that the oil came from the very first press of the olives, and typically no chemicals are used in that process. Choose oils that are fresh and store them in a cool, dark place. When oils are exposed to light, oxygen, or heat they can quickly become rancid. You'll know they have gone bad when they smell fishy or like Play-doh. Once they have been oxidized, they are rancid and unhealthy for consumption. If that occurs, toss them out and buy some fresh oils for your home.

Plant Foods

Plant foods are beans, peas, lentils, vegetables, fruits, grains, nuts, seeds, and squashes. Plant foods are naturally rich in nutrients and fiber and contain no cholesterol. Most people have a few favorite plant foods that they eat on a regular basis, so finding your favorites will help you make them a part of your daily diet. Keeping a bowl of fresh fruit or chopped up vegetables encourages us to grab a healthy snack when we're busy. Also making dishes ahead of time is quite helpful to healthy nourishment; for example, preparing a lentil soup or vegetable chili on the weekend to have on hand during a busy workweek is a habit that will save you money and time during the week. Having the right foods available for our meals or for whenever we're hungry is the best way to stick to a healthy diet.

Making your own protein bars with whole oats, barley malt syrup, and soy flour could save you a lot of money, and you can make them with your favorite nuts, sunflower seeds, dried fruits, or even a handful of organic, naturally sweetened chocolate chips. You can also replace the fat and sugar with healthier alternatives so that your personally designed protein bars can have all the ingredients you need to keep your energy up, keep you burning fat, and even satisfy your sweet tooth.

Nutrient-Dense Foods

Some foods have so many vitamins and minerals that they are almost a dietary supplement; such foods include seaweeds and nutritional yeast. Seaweeds include nori, hijiki, arame, kombu, and dulse and have many minerals from the ocean water. Use the nori to make sushi, buy seaweed salads that just need water to reconstitute, and try adding a piece of kombu to your soups to add flavor and nutrients. One easy way to get seaweed nutrients is to get a bottle of dried seaweed seasoning and add a sprinkle to your grain dishes or to top off your salad.

Nutritional yeast contains high amounts of B vitamins and some trace minerals as well. It's a cheesy-tasting dried product that comes in flakes or powder. It tastes great on popcorn, on corn tortillas with a little butter, and in macaroni and cheese.

Shopping Tips

There are several co-ops and healthy markets across the country such as Whole Foods Markets, Wild Oats, Fresh Fields, New Frontier, and Trader Joe's where you will find everything from steel-cut oats and extra virgin olive oil to seaweeds and nutritional yeast, plus organic baked chips, wheat-free and dairy-free products, and loads more. It's all about healthy choices, and you won't go hungry. There are many more in my book, *The Staying Healthy Shopper's Guide.* Our Resource section has other good ideas and contacts.

Physical Support During Your Transition

As you start incorporating more physical activity into your daily routine, you will increase your caloric needs. So do this slowly and gently over a two-week period to give your body time to adjust. Yoga and stretching will help awaken your body after your cleanse (and during as well) and assist in the last stage of cleansing. Deep stretching massages the internal organs helping to move out old fluids and bring in fresh blood containing nutrients and oxygen. Also continuing with steams, Epsom salt baths, and dry brushing of the skin will help your body release those deeper layers of toxins through the completion phase of your detoxification program.

THE TRANSITIONAL DIETS

The Hypoallergenic, Long-Term Detox Diet

Those who have been diagnosed with food allergies or sensitivities or those suspecting they may be suffering from any food reactions can now test their hypothesis. After cleansing you can assess how you respond to individual foods by reintroducing them one at a time. Even if you have not considered that you may have food reactions, you may have had mystery symptoms that disappeared during your cleanse. In this case, you should take advantage of this transition phase to test for possible reactive foods.

Transitioning back to a more normal diet after you have finished your cleanse should be done in steps. Many people are reactive to common foods such as wheat, dairy, soy, sugar, peanuts, corn, and eggs—The Sensitive Seven. Wait for a while before you reintroduce these. Later you can retest those foods to see if they weaken your health. Add them in one by one, and not more than one every day or two.

A brief review of my book, *The False Fat Diet,* and the Sensitive Seven Elimination Plan will give you the general idea. This eating plan is one of the most popular with patients because they usually feel better and lose weight; it eliminates all of the seven most commonly reactive foods: dairy products, wheat, corn, eggs, soy, peanuts, and sugar. If you are also reactive to foods other than the Sensitive Seven, such as tomatoes, potatoes, or oranges, you might want to eliminate them as well. In addition, you

SAMPLE MENU: HYPOALLEGENIC DIET

Day 1

Breakfast:
- Hot Steel-Cut Oats,* with 1–2 teaspoons honey (or maple syrup) and 2 tablespoons rice milk (small 4–6 ounce bowl)
- Fruit salad (6-ounce bowl with banana, apple, raisins)
- Hot herbal tea

Snack:
- Rice crackers or rice bread with 1 tablespoon almond butter or 1 tablespoon all-fruit spread
- Fruit juice (8-ounce glass)

Lunch:
- Tuna salad, with sliced celery or onion and 1–2 tablespoons vinaigrette dressing
- Steamed and seasoned green beans (½ cup)
- Spelt or rice bread (1 slice), with 1 teaspoon almond butter or fruit spread

Snack:
- Carrot and celery sticks (5–10)
- Almonds (5–10) or sunflower seeds (20–40 or 1 handful)

Dinner:
- Stuffed Bell Pepper* or Herbed Soup* (12-ounce bowl)
- Green salad with 1 tablespoon vinaigrette dressing
- Iced herbal tea

Snack:
- Pears in Black Cherry Juice* or a piece of fruit

Day 2

Breakfast:
- Hot Breakfast Quinoa* and Baked Apples*
- Hot herbal tea

Snack:
- Apple
- Walnuts

Lunch:
- Gazpacho* and Pea Hummus*
- Iced herb tea

Snack:
- Rice crackers (or other snack from Chapter 13)

Dinner:
- Vegetable Curry* or Lentil Stew*
- Glazed broccoli
- Green salad with Ginger Garlic Dressing*

Snack:
- Baked Apple, with cinnamon raisins and 1 teaspoon honey

*Recipes can be found in chater 13.

should eliminate any food that you have been eating most every day or foods that you crave.

Your loss of water weight and adipose tissue in this eating plan will depend upon several factors. Among the most important is your activity level. If you are very active and exercise an hour or more each day, you may lose several pounds a week. If you are moderately active and exercise every other day, you may lose a pound or two each week. If you are inactive and don't exercise at all, you may not lose weight at all and might even gradually gain some weight. In addition, men will tend to lose adipose tissue on this eating plan more quickly than women, because men generally have a higher percentage of muscle and usually burn fat more efficiently.

Another factor that will determine your rate of weight loss is your size. Both men and women lose weight more quickly the more overweight they are. If you are a very heavy person, you will tend to lose more weight on this eating plan than a small, lighter person. If you are inactive, or if you are a woman, you may need to eat somewhat less food than this eating plan calls for, in order to lose weight. You can do this by reducing your portion sizes or avoiding some of the foods the plan calls for.

After at least one week on this eating plan, you may begin to reintroduce suspected reactive foods as you begin your food "challenges." You could also add puréed vegetable soups or a "cream" of vegetable soup blended with a very loose oatmeal instead of dairy. Another idea is to eat a lighter lunch or dinner on some days or just drink juice at those times.

The Detox Doc's Anti-Candida Diet

If you have been diagnosed with Candida or other yeast overgrowth, you will want to continue to avoid simple sugars (and alcohol and vinegars) even after you transition back to a long-term program. Avoid sugar, refined flours, and excessive use of natural sweeteners such as honey, maple syrup, fruit juice, turbinado sugar, and so forth. The bulk of your diet should be composed of vegetables, beans, peas, lentils, fish, nuts and seeds, olive oil, and to a lesser degree whole grains and high-quality meats.

The overall approach to treating the yeast problem is threefold. The first facet is to refrain from feeding those "yeastie beasties" what they like to eat, so they can't thrive and divide. They live on mostly simple sugars, yeast, and fermented foods. These include fruits, fruit juices, and dried fruits, sugary foods, refined flour products, alcoholic beverages, cheese, vinegar, breads, and other yeasted fermented food products, such as soy sauce. All these foods are avoided on the yeast diet.

What to eat? There are many recommended foods—fish, poultry, meat, lots of vegetables, some whole grains, nuts, seeds, and occasional eggs. (The anti-yeast diet is more difficult for vegetarians, but definitely possible.) Some yogurt, especially acidophilus culture, is all right if milk is tolerated. Oils are obtained from the nuts and seeds, as well as from some butter and more cold-pressed vegetable oils, such as olive, flaxseed, sesame, and sunflower. Legumes are often limited because they add to intestinal gas. Initially, the diet includes no fruit, or only one piece a day, and none of the sweeter fruits, such as grapes, bananas, and melons.

Basic meals include proteins and vegetables or, occasionally, starch and vegetables. For the first few weeks, the starches and carbohydrates, including pastas and especially breads, are limited to one to two portions daily, mainly as whole-grain cereals. This includes some brown rice, millet, oatmeal, or corn polenta. Reducing starchy foods does lower the fiber intake, but usually other aspects of the treatment help colon function. The Anti-Yeast Diet, discussed next, can also be used to reduce yeast and parasites.

The anti-yeast diet is a special therapeutic diet, and not necessarily a lifelong one, although many people like the way they feel on it. Intestinal symptoms decrease, energy improves, and itchy or irritated skin may start to heal with a decrease in sugar and yeasty foods. Also, some weight can be shed easily on this diet. This may be a problem for the already trim person, and lighter people need to emphasize regular eating to prevent weight loss, including more nuts and seeds and nut butters especially.

After a few weeks, we can test ourselves with fruit, bread, other grain products, or cheese—of course, one food at a time, and only one new one daily—to see how we handle them. If they seem to cause no problems, we can then bring these foods into our diet on a rotating basis, like every few days. Eventually, adding more whole grains and fiber will provide what I believe is a healthier diet. Different degrees of strictness with the diet may be necessary, depending on the severity of the problem and the individual. A more stringent diet might exclude all fruits; whole grains, particularly the glutinous ones—wheat, barley, rye, and oats; herb teas and spices, which may contain molds; and many nuts, which can also carry molds.

ANTI-YEAST DIET PLAN

Emphasize		Avoid	
Vegetables—all	Beans	Sugar—all forms	Baked goods
Meats*	Nuts & seeds	Alcoholic beverages	Vinegars
Poultry*	Butter	Fruit juices	Pickled vegetables
Eggs	Cold-pressed oils	Dried fruits	Cheese
Fish*	Lemon	Refined flours	Mushrooms
Whole grains	Fresh fruit**	Breads	

* Vegetarians will need to use more whole grains, beans, and nuts and seeds, but this higher carbohydrate diet does not really curb yeast as well. Furthermore, vegetarians seem to be more prone to yeast overgrowth because their diet is more alkaline and sweet, which supports the yeast. Yeast does not grow as well in an acid environment, and thus many of the anti-yeast herbs and medicines are fairly acidic.
**Limit to two pieces daily.

Other facets of a good anti-yeast program involve intake of healthy bacteria and probiotics, such as *Lactobacillus acidophilus* and *Bifidobacteria*. These help to reduce growth and provide what our colon wants. Also, take herbs and medicines that help to kill or inhibit the yeast growth. These include such natural supplements as garlic, grapefruit seed extract, oregano oil, plant tannins, caprylic acid, undecylenic acid, and berberine (a goldenseal herb extract). Most of these substances can be a little irritating.

If garlic is used, take two capsules several times daily. Pau d'arco, a Brazilian tree bark, and other plant tannins are popular herbs in the treatment of yeast, allergies, and other immune problems. They can be taken in capsules, or tea made from the bark can be drunk several times daily. It seems to tone or strengthen the gastrointestinal tract and may help reduce yeast. Caprylic acid is popular; however, in sensitivity tests it doesn't appear to be very effective in eradicating the yeast. I often use short courses of systemic drugs to really clear Candida and other yeasts. The most common one I prescribe is Nizoral (ketoconazole), and then Diflucan (fluconazole), and Sporanox (itraconoazale) and nystatin less commonly. The effects of nystatin have lessened over the years. These systemic drugs can cause some liver irritation, yet most people tolerate them well, and with stopping, the liver clears easily. I often have people use milk thistle (silymarin) herb, about 60 to 80 mg twice daily. Doing the whole program is the best way to clear Candida-related problems. I refer you to Chapter 17 in my book, *Staying Healthy with Nutrition,* for a more complete discussion.

Staying Healthy After Detox: A Vital Diet for Life

The Detox Diet book and *A Cookbook for All Seasons* have always been companions in practice. My patients often use one and then the other. In fact, the original Detox Diet, with the fruit and whole grain in the morning and the steamed vegetables at lunch and dinner, is the skeleton, or the basic structure, of the seasonal menu plans from my cookbook.

The Detox Diet program as you have in this book is not a completely balanced eating plan for the long term. It tends to be too low in protein and even calories, and could benefit from the good essential oils found in raw nuts and seeds. *A Cookbook for All Seasons,* is complete and one of the healthiest lifelong eating plans.

The sample diet (see pages 98 and 99) shows a chart with the daily balance and combination of foods over the day. As with The Detox Diet, we start with two glasses of water first thing, maybe with a half a lemon squeezed in one to stimulate the digestion. That's followed by a piece or two of fruit, which is followed by some starch, such as a whole-grain cereal. Then we add a handful of nuts or seeds mid-morning to get our digestion going even more. For lunch we suggest a salad or cooked vegetables with some protein, such as a piece of poultry or some sprouted beans for a vegetarian. A mid-afternoon snack can be another piece of fruit or some veggies. If you wish more calories, it can be a rice cake or two with some almond butter. Dinner is more vegetables (remember, they're the most important) with a starch or a protein. We are food-combining, which doesn't mix starch and proteins. If you are still working to reduce weight, the less starch the better. Meals of veggies and protein are best for that purpose. There is an optional evening light snack, such as popcorn or an apple and a date. And if you have a good date (pun intended), and he or she is interesting, you can be occupied, enjoy nature and each other, and not think about food.

This is an ideal diet, especially if you eat only seasonal, local, and organic foods. *A Cookbook for All Seasons* offers the whole story as we move through the year, with seasonal food selections and recipes. Finding what's available at the time of year—in your garden, store, or farmer' market—and then creating your menu from that, is a healthy way to think about cooking, rather than picking a recipe and going out to find those specific foods. That's what the great European chefs are known for. Remember, fresh is best, organic is ideal, and your health is the most important commodity to an enjoyable life.

AFTER DETOX MENU PLAN

Day One

Fruit and/or Juice:	Organic Apple or Energizing Elixir* fresh juice
Breakfast:	Hot Breakfast Quinoa*
Lunch:	White Bean Salad* and fresh Harvest Juice*
Snack:	Cold Almonds*
Dinner:	Salmon with Roasted Garlic and Rosemary*
Treat:	Juice Jells*

Keep a food journal. Check the recipes and seasonal ideas that are your favorites and keep them for later motivation and tastes.

Day Two

Fruit and/or Juice:	Organic Grapes or Sunset Soother* fresh juice
Breakfast:	Baked Apple*
Lunch:	Herbed Soup*
Snack:	Cottonwood Pea Hummus*
Dinner:	Kombu Squash Soup*
Treat:	Fresh fruit juice or smoothie of your choice

Day Three

Fruit:	Grapefruit or After-Workout Refresher* fresh juice
Breakfast:	Basic Breakfast Steel Cut Oats*
Lunch:	Jicama Salad* and Gazpacho*
Snack:	Kombu Knots*
Dinner:	Glazed Broccoli* and Lentil Stew*
Treat:	Pears in Black Cherry Sauce*

Feeling better? Of course! Several healthy courses are coursing through you now, healing your body and blood, and giving you future interest in your health bank account.

Day Four

Fruit:	Cantaloupe or Tobin's Strawberry Almond Shake*
Breakfast:	Breakfast Rice* with nuts and raisins
Lunch:	Quick Southwest Quinoa*
Snack:	Fresh juice or smoothie of your choice
Dinner:	Vegetable Curry* with Date and Orange Chutney*
Treat:	Baked Apple*

Day Five

Fruit:	Purple Papaya Smoothie*
Breakfast:	Breakfast Millet* or Baked Apples
Lunch:	Stuffed Bell Peppers* and green salad with Ginger Garlic Dressing*
Snack:	Asian Cucumber Salad* and Carrot Cocktail*
Dinner:	Broccoli Soup* and Caramelized Onion Quinoa*
Treat:	Cold Almonds and Cinnamon Cider

By now, you have some recipe ideas of your own. Enjoy these good flavors and the new foods you are choosing to consume.

Day Six

Fruit:	Pears and Apple Lemonade Juice*
Breakfast:	Dani's Muesli*
Lunch:	Herbed Millet* with Steamed Vegetables
Snack:	Guacamole* with baby carrots
Dinner:	Caraway Cabbage Borscht*
Treat:	Gingered Green Tea* or Banana Soother* smoothie

*These recipes are included in Chapter 13.

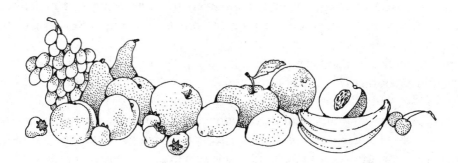

CHAPTER SIX

Supplements for Detoxification

♦

There are many aspects to healthy detoxification. It is important to support all the organs that help us to detoxify—the skin, kidneys, colon, liver, and lungs. Drinking water is crucial to flush toxins. Regular exercise and sweating is also important, as is lymphatic massage. And keeping our bowels moving is necessary to feeling well during detox programs.

Colon cleansing is one of the most important steps in detoxification. The large intestine releases many toxins, and sluggish functioning of this organ can rapidly produce general toxicity. During any detox program, most people will incorporate some colon cleansing. Helpful products include laxatives, fiber, and colon detox supplements such as psyllium seed husks alone or mixed with other agents (such as aloe vera powder, bentonite clay, and acidophilus culture). Enemas using water, herbs, or even diluted coffee (stimulates liver cleansing, and although popular in some detox programs, I do not recommend) may be used. A series of colonic water irrigations (best performed by a trained professional with filtered water and sterile equipment) can be the focal point of a detox program accompanied by a cleansing diet and fiber supplements.* Whatever the method, keeping the bowels moving is key to feeling well during detoxification.

Regular exercise is also very important during detox (as always) as it stimulates sweating and encourages elimination through the skin. Exercise also improves our general metabolism and helps overall with detoxification. For this reason, regular aerobic exercise is key to maintaining a nontoxic body, especially when we indulge in various substances such as sugar or alcohol. Since exercise releases toxins in the body, it is important to incorporate adequate fluids, antioxidants, vitamins, and minerals.

Regular bathing cleanses the skin of toxins that have been released and opens the pores for further elimination, and are particularly beneficial during detoxification.

---

* There are many herbal and fiber programs for colon detoxification available, found mainly in health food stores. For a complete body and colon cleansing program, I really like Nature's Pure Body Program available through their toll-free number (800) 952-7873. Check out my website www.elsonhaas.com for other contacts.

Saunas and sweats are commonly used to enhance skin elimination. Dry brushing the skin with an appropriate skin brush before bathing is also suggested to invigorate the skin and cleanse away old cells. Massage therapy (especially lymphatic or deep massage) stimulates elimination and body functions and promotes relaxation. Clearing generalized tensions also makes for a more complete detoxification.

Resting, relaxation, and recharging are also important to this rejuvenation process. During the detox process, we may need more rest, quiet time, and sleep, although most commonly we have more energy and function better on less sleep than before. Relaxation exercises help our body rebalance itself as our mind and attitudes stop interfering with our natural homeostasis. The practice of yoga combines quiet yet powerful exercises with breath awareness and regulation, allowing increased flexibility and relaxation.

Certain supplements are appropriate for some detoxification programs. However, general supplementation may be less important in this detox program than with the specific detox plans for alcohol, caffeine, and nicotine, when more nutrients can ease withdrawal symptoms. *(These specific substance detoxification programs are discussed in later chapters.)* For straight juice cleansing or water fasts, we usually do not recommend very many supplements; however, some nutrients or herbs to stimulate the detoxification process may be helpful. Examples include potassium, extra fiber with olive oil to clear toxins from the colon, sodium alginate from seaweeds to bind heavy metals, and apple cider vinegar in water (1 tablespoon vinegar in 8 ounces hot water) to help reduce mucus. Blue-green algae, chlorella, and spirulina are nutrient-rich foods that may supply physical and mental energy. For people who begin with transition diets, a specialized nutrient program may help neutralize toxins and support elimination. With weight loss (for detoxers who are overweight), toxins stored in the fat will need to be mobilized and cleared—more water, fiber, and antioxidant nutrients can help handle this.

The supplement program used for general detoxification (with additional support to reduce nutrient deficiency during detox) is outlined in the table at the end of this chapter. It includes a low-dosage multiple vitamin/mineral supplement to fulfill the basic nutritional requirements during the transitional diet. The B vitamins, particularly niacin, are also important, as are minerals such as zinc, calcium, magnesium, and potassium. The antioxidant nutrients include vitamins C and E, beta-carotene or mixed carotenoids, vitamin A, zinc, and selenium. Some authorities believe that higher amounts of vitamin A (10,000 IU), mixed carotenoids (25,000 to 50,000 IU), vitamin C (8 to 12 g), selenium (300 to 400 mcg), and vitamin E (1,000 to 1,200 IU) are helpful during detoxification to neutralize the free radicals.

The liver is our most important detoxification organ. The B vitamins, especially B_3 (niacin) and B_6 (pyridoxine), vitamins A and C, zinc, calcium, vitamin E and selenium, and L-cysteine are all also needed to support liver detoxification. Milk thistle herb (often sold as silymarin or *Silybum marianum*) has also been shown to aid liver detoxification and repair.

Several amino acids improve or support detoxification, particularly cysteine and methionine, which contain sulfur. L-cysteine supplies sulfhydryl groups, which help prevent oxidation and bind heavy metals such as mercury; vitamin C and selenium aid this process as well. Cysteine is the precursor to glutathione—our most important detoxifier—which counters many chemicals and carcinogens. Glutathione is synthesized to form detoxification enzymes *glutathione peroxidase* and *reductase,* which work to prevent peroxidation of lipids and to decrease toxins such as smoke, radiation, auto exhaust, chemicals, drugs, and other carcinogens.

Glycine is a secondary helper. An amino acid that supports glutathione synthesis, glycine decreases the toxicity of substances such as phenols or benzoic acid (a food

---

SIMPLE SUPPLEMENTS FOR THE NEW DETOX DIET

- Multivitamin/mineral (one-a-day type)
  One tablet or capsule after breakfast

- Antioxidant combination
  1–2 caps or tabs twice daily, between meals

- Vitamin C or buffered powdered C with minerals (calcium, magnesium, and potassium)
  One tab or cap of 500-1,000 mg Vitamin C, or ½–1 teaspoon twice daily of powder mixed into liquid

- Calcium-magnesium capsule or tablet
  1–3 caps at bedtime or 1–2 for any muscle cramps to be utilized if the buffered vitamin C powder is not being used

- Blue-green algae, spirulina, or chlorella
  2–4 tabs or caps after breakfast and lunch (double the number of tabs for chlorella because they are smaller)

- Herbal colon tablets of laxative tea
  1–2 tabs twice daily in the morning and evening, or about ½–1 cup of tea, morning and evening (varies depending on individual sensitivity)

- Herbal extracts can also be used to support or balance other body systems or to enhance energy. Siberian or other ginsengs are possible, echinacea for immune support, ginger for circulation, etc. *Review the organized lists of herbs later in this chapter.*

preservative). Glutamine is also important in helping to heal the GI tract as well as reduce cravings for sugar and alcohol, should they occur. Other amino acids that may have mild detoxifying effects are methionine, tyrosine, and taurine.*

As mentioned earlier, fiber also supports detoxification. Psyllium seed husks (often combined with other detox nutrients, such as pectin, aloe vera, alginates, and/or colon herbs) help cleanse mucus along the small intestine, create bulk in the colon, and pull toxins from the gastrointestinal tract. When fiber is combined with one or two table-spoons of olive oil, it helps bind toxins and reduce the absorption of fats and some basic minerals. Psyllium husks also reduce absorption of the olive oil itself, which is important in reducing calories and binding any fat-soluble chemicals that may have been released. An option then involves taking 1 to 2 teaspoons each of psyllium husks and bran several times daily (with meals and at bedtime) along with one teaspoon of olive oil to help detoxify the colon. Acidophilus and other beneficial bacteria (pro-biotics) in the colon neutralize some toxins, reduce the metabolism of other microbes, and lessen colon toxicity. Supplemental probiotics can be added to the detox program.

WATER

Remember, water is crucial to any type of detox program for diluting and eliminating toxin accumulations. It is probably our most important detoxifier as it helps us clean through our skin and kidneys, and improves our sweating with exercise. One of my favorite sayings is, "Dilution is the solution to pollution." Eight to ten glasses a day (depending on body size and activity level) of clean, filtered water are suggested. Some authorities suggest using distilled water during detox programs, as its lack of minerals draws other particles (nutrients and toxins) to it. Distilled water throws off our biochemical/electrical balance, and so regular, purified or clean spring water are preferred. Two or three glasses of water thirty to sixty minutes before each meal (and at night) will help flush toxins during our body's natural elimination time.

Water Tips and Stats

- Lack of water is the primary cause of daytime *fatigue and headaches.*
- 75 percent of Americans are *chronically* dehydrated, particularly the elderly.
- The thirst mechanism is often so weak that it can be *mistaken for hunger.*
- Even *mild* dehydration will slow down one's metabolism by as much as 3 percent, and more severe dehydration by 5 percent.

* For more information on amino acid metabolism and uses, review Chapter 3, Proteins, from my book, *Staying Healthy with Nutrition.*

- One glass of water stopped midnight *hunger pangs* for almost all of the dieters studied in a University of Washington study.
- Preliminary research indicates that 8 to 10 glasses of water a day could significantly *ease back and joint pain* for up to 80 percent of sufferers.
- A mere 2 percent drop in body water can trigger *fuzzy short-term memory, trouble with basic math,* and *difficulty focusing* on the computer screen or on a printed page.

How Much Water Should You Drink?

There is some controversy on how much we really need daily, but we think it's healthy to drink at least two quarts, which is sixty-four ounces or eight 8-ounce glasses. Yet, read on to see all the important factors in determining how much water you really need.

Drying Effects

Many factors affect your bodies need for water. You may need more or less drinking water depending on lifestyle, diet, medications, and so forth. For example, if you eat a lot of drying foods such as breads, crackers, salty foods, and high-fat or sugary foods, you will need more water just to process these foods through your digestive system. Also if you take in caffeine and other diuretics such as coffee, espresso, tea (black and green), chocolate, or caffeinated sodas (such as Coke, Pepsi, or Mountain Dew), you are flushing water and electrolytes out of your system and must replace that fluid and nutrients. Many lifestyle choices can be drying, such as drinking alcohol (wine, beer, and hard alcohol), smoking, recreational drugs and OTC (over the counter) drugs, chewing tobacco, and cigars. Also, if your environment is dry because you use high heat in your house or car or heavy blankets at night then you will have an increased need for water.

Hydrating Habits

On the other hand, if you eat a lot of fresh fruits and vegetables and drink high-water-content juices and other liquids, such as almond and other nut milks, soy milk, or rice milk, your daily need for water will be lower. Eating cooked whole grains and legumes add some further hydration; legumes are beans, peas, and lentils. They are full of beneficial soluble fiber such as gels and pectins that help hold onto water in your intestines, allowing your body to reabsorb water before it passes through you. Also EFAs (essential fatty acids) from fish and plants, such as flax and borage, are important dietary nutrients for water absorption into the cells.

Athlete's Water Needs

Most people sweat when they work out and lose a considerable amount of water and electrolytes through their pores. A general guideline for water replacement is one quart of electrolyte water (thirty-two ounces) for every hour of heavy exercise. That includes hiking, running, swimming, lifting weights, tennis, yard work, cleaning house, and so forth.

What Are Electrolytes?

Potassium, magnesium, sodium, calcium, and chloride are electrical conductors necessary for nerve and heart function, as well as supporting hydration.

Electrolyte Replacement Drinks

Don't fall for those inferior sugary, chemical-food colored mixes such as Gatorade. There are several high-quality electrolyte drinks and powder mixes now available. Knudsen makes an electrolyte replacement drink called Recharge, which is a mix of fruit juice, water, and electrolytes. It is available in orange, lemon, and fruit punch flavors. Alacer Corporation makes the popular Emergen-C products and an inexpensive electrolyte powder called Electro-Mix. This product contains no food coloring, sugar, or calories.

Natural Electrolyte Replacement

Fruits and vegetables are rich in natural electrolytes. Drink smoothies, fresh fruit juices, or buy bottled or canned concentrate of organic fruit juices. Also, nuts and seeds contain loads of nutrients, and they do have good oils (and calories), so eating a handful or so provides good fuel for activity or recharging after exercise.

Niacin-Sauna Therapy

A special detoxification process has been developed to help in the release of chemicals, pesticides, and pharmaceutical drugs, many of which are stored more deeply in the body fat, tissues, and organs. Used in some clinics, this program includes several weeks of a high-fluid and juice diet, exercise, and a high intake of niacin (vitamin B$_3$) with sauna therapy. The extended saunas may last several hours, with breaks to drink fluids. Niacin is a vasostimulator and vasodilator, aiding circulation. The idea is to cleanse hidden chemicals from fat and other body tissues through juice cleansing, weight loss, niacin therapy, exercise, and sweats. The new infra-red saunas are acceptable.

The niacin-sauna program has therapeutic possibilities as an intense, medically supervised detoxification process; however, it is still experimental and does entail risks.

Preliminary results are good—especially for people with symptoms caused by exposure to herbicides such as Agent Orange—yet there are some drawbacks. The program is costly and time-consuming. This extreme detox can also cause nutrient deficiencies that can take months to replenish. Proper nutrient restoration must be ensured, both during and after this therapy. This program does help detoxification from many chemicals and drugs (especially the recreational types) and from daily abuses of alcohol and nicotine. Many of us can do a modified version of this therapy on our own with sauna, the newer infra-red saunas, a few days of juice cleansing, regular exercise, and supplemental niacin (beginning at 100 to 200 mg and moving up to 2 to 3 grams daily). Be sure to replenish fluids and minerals. *If you have any pre-existing medical problems, weakness, or fatigue, see a physician first.*

Note: You *do* want the simple, inexpensive niacin that causes flushing and not the fancier flush-free inositol hexanicotinate.

CLEANSING HERBS

Garlic—blood cleanser, may lower blood fats and cholesterol, natural antibiotic/antimicrobial for bacteria, yeasts, parasites, and viral infections

Red clover blossoms—blood cleanser, good during convalescence and healing

Echinacea—lymph cleanser, improves lymphocyte and phagocyte actions, immunity supporter, antimicrobial

Dandelion root—liver and blood cleanser, diuretic, filters toxins, a tonic

Chaparral—strong blood cleanser, with possibilities for use in cancer therapy

Cayenne pepper—blood and tissue purifier, increases fluid elimination and sweat, a natural stimulant

Cascara sagrada—a colon cleanser and bowel tonic

Ginger root—stimulates circulation and sweating, relieves congestion, help nausea

Licorice root—the "great detoxifier," biochemical balancer, mild laxative, supports immune function, stomach soother (for inflammation/irritation)

Yellow dock root—skin, blood, and liver cleanser, contains vitamin C and iron

Burdock root—skin and blood cleanser, diuretic and diaphoretic (increases perspiration), improves liver function, antibacterial and antifungal properties

Sarsaparilla root—blood and lymph cleanser, contains saponins, which reduce microbes and toxins, used in making root beer

Prickly ash bark—good for nerves and joints, anti-infectious

Oregon grape root—skin and colon cleanser, blood purifier, liver stimulant

Parsley leaf—diuretic, flushes kidneys, green purifier, and breath freshener

Goldenseal root—blood, liver, kidney, and skin cleanser, stimulates detoxification, antimicrobial

A GENERAL CLASSIFICATION OF HERBS USEFUL IN DETOXIFICATION*

Blood Cleansers
Echinacea
Red clover
Dandelion
Burdock
Yellow dock
Oregon grape root

Laxatives/Colon Cleansers
Cascara sagrada
Buckthorn
Dandelion
Yellow dock
Rhubarb root
Senna leaf
Licorice

Diuretics
Parsley
Yarrow
Cleavers
Horsetail
Corn silk
Uva ursi
Juniper berries

Skin Cleansers (Diaphoretics)**
Burdock
Oregon grape
Yellow dock
Goldenseal
Boneset
Elder flowers
Peppermint
Cayenne pepper
Ginger root

Antibiotics
Garlic
Myrrh
Prickly ash
Wormwood
Echinacea
Propolis
Clove
Eucalyptus

Anticatarrhals***
Echinacea
Boneset
Goldenseal
Sage
Hyssop
Garlic
Yarrow

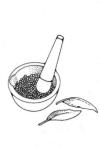

* Not usually used with fasting or juice cleansing, but as supplements to dietary detoxification—using herbs alone may be the most productive in some detoxification programs. A program that includes juice cleansing and specific herbal therapies is best designed by an experienced practitioner in natural medicine and detoxification.
** Diaphoretics increase perspiration
*** Anticatarrhals help eliminate mucus.

SAMPLE DETOX FORMULA

Echinacea
Goldenseal root
Yellow dock root

Cayenne pepper
Garlic

Parsley leaf
Licorice root

Obtain powders (or ground herbs) in equal amounts for all of the above except cayenne, for which you should get half. Mix and put into "00" capsules. Take two capsules, two or three times daily between meals. Drink lots of water with this as well.

GENERAL DETOXIFICATION NUTRIENT PROGRAM

The following program has ranges on most nutrients and supplies the body with the vitamins and minerals, amino and fatty acids that support our tissues, our healthy liver as well as the overall process of detoxification. See page 102 for specific programs for Detox Diet.

GENERAL DETOXIFICATION NUTRIENT PROGRAM—DAILY AMOUNTS

Water	2 ½–3 qt	Biotin	200 mcg
Fiber	20-40 g	Vitamin C	1–4 g
Vitamin A	4,000–6,000 IU	Bioflavonoids	250–500 mg
Beta-carotene or mixed carotenoids	15,000–30,000 IU	Calcium	600–850 mg
		Chromium	200 mcg
Vitamin D	200–400 IU	Copper	2 mg
Vitamin E	400–1,000 IU	Iodine	150 mcg
Vitamin K	200 mcg	Magnesium	300–500 mg
Thiamine (B_1)	10–25 mg	Manganese	5–10 mg
Riboflavin (B_2)	10–25 mg	Molybdenum	300 mcg
Niacinamide (B_3)	50 mg	Potassium	300-500 mg
Niacin (B_3)	50–2,000 mg*	Selenium	300 mcg
Pantothenic acid (B_5)	250–500 mg	Silicon	100 mg
Pyridoxine (B_6)	10–25 mg	Vanadium	300 mcg
Cobalamin (B_{12})	50–100 mcg	Zinc	30 mg
Folic acid	400–800 mcg		

OPTIONAL

L-amino acids (general blend)	500–1,000 mg	Extra virgin olive oil	3–6 teaspoons
L-cysteine	500–1,000 mg	Liquid chlorophyll	2–4 teaspoons
DL-methionine	250–500 mg	Apple cider vinegar	1–2 tablespoons
L-glycine	250–500 mg		
L-glutamine	500–1,000 mg		
Psyllium seed	2–4 teaspoons or 8–12 caps		
Flaxseed oil	1–2 teaspoons or 2–4 caps		
Acidophilus/Probiotic culture,	more than 2 billion organisms/day		
Detox formula herbs:	4–6 capsules		

echinacea, yellow dock, goldenseal, garlic, parsley, licorice, cayenne pepper

*May be used for special detox programs; see page 105–106.

CHAPTER SEVEN

Sugar Detoxification

For most of us, sugar is a symbol of love and nurturance because as infants, our first food is lactose, or milk sugar. Overconsumption and daily use of sugar is the first compulsive habit for most everyone with addictions later in life. Simple sugar, or glucose, is what our body, our cells, and brain use as fuel for energy. Some glucose is stored in our liver and muscle tissues as glycogen for future use; excess sugar is stored as fat for use during periods of low-calorie intake or starvation.

Problems with sweets come from the frequency with which we eat them and the quantity of sugar we consume. The type of sugar we eat is also a contributing factor. Refined sugar or sucrose (a disaccharide made up of two sugars—glucose and fructose) is usually extracted from sugar cane or sugar beets, initially whole foods. However, most all of the nutrients are removed and retained only in the discarded extract called molasses. When the manufacturing process is complete, the result is pure sugar, a refined crystal that contains four calories per gram and essentially no nutrients.

Sugar and sweeteners have so pervaded our food manufacturing and restaurant industries that it is almost impossible to find prepackaged products that are unsweetened. Most frequently used are both refined, high-calorie, non-nutrient sucrose and the corn syrup derivatives, mainly as high-fructose corn syrup. Consequently, the only way to avoid sweeteners is to avoid packaged products and recipes with sugar whenever possible. Fruits contain natural fructose, in balance with other nutrients; honey and maple syrup are more highly concentrated natural sugars and are appropriate for most of us in moderation.

Traditional Chinese medicine views the desire for sugar, or the sweet flavor, as a craving for the mother (yin) energy, a craving that represents a need for comfort or security. A desire for spicy or salty flavored foods might represent looking for the father (yang) energy or power and direction. In Western cultures, we have turned sugar into a reward system (a tangible symbol of material nurturing) to the degree that many of us have been conditioned to need some sweet treat to feel complete or satisfied. We continue these patterns with our children, unconsciously showing our affection for them by giving them sugary foods. Holidays and special occasions are centered around sugar—birthday cakes and ice cream, Halloween candy, chocolate Easter eggs, Thanksgiving pie, Christmas cookies, Valentine chocolates—the list is endless. We even reward our children for good behavior by giving them treats. Sweet talk is embedded in our language—sweetie, sweetie pie, sweetheart, honey, honey pie, sugar, sugar baby, candy, sweet cakes, baby cakes, honey bun, sugar plum, and so on. The message is loud and clear: sweetness=love.

SUGAR AND HEALTH

Many nutritional authorities feel that the high use of sugar in our diet is a significant underlying cause of disease. Too much sweetener in any form can have a negative effect on our health; this includes not only refined sugar, but also corn syrup, honey, fruit juices, and treats such as sodas, cakes, and candies. Because sugary foods satisfy our hunger, they often replace more nutritious foods and weaken our tissue's health and disease resistance.

PROBLEMS ASSOCIATED WITH SUGAR INTAKE*

Tooth decay

Obesity and its increased risk of **diabetes, cancer,** and other diseases

Nutritional deficiency—including anemia, protein and mineral deficiencies

Hypoglycemia and carbohydrate imbalance

Chronic dyspepsia and digestive problems

Immune dysfunction and problems such as recurrent infections

Menstrual irregularities & premenstrual symptoms (PMS)

Yeast overgrowth and its many subsequent problems, including craving sweets and carbohydrates

Hyperactivity and difficulty concentrating

Alcoholism—a potential link as it is associated with hypoglycemia and abnormal carbohydrate metabolism

Mood swings, anxiety, depression

Heart disease

*There is much evidence that eating too many sweets eventually causes disease. If these conditions occur in either your personal or family history, it is important to seriously consider a dietary change for your health's sake.

Sugar can also compromise our body's ability to fight illness. In 1976, Emanuel Cheraskin, MD, and others showed that a single intake of sugar can lower the bacteria-fighting capabilities of white blood cells (phagocytic activity) in the blood of test subjects for up to five hours. In a number of other studies, researchers found a positive correlation between sugar overconsumption and eight forms of cancer—colon, rectum, breast, ovary, prostate, kidney, nervous system, and pancreas. In some cases, the risk was more than doubled by consuming sugar on a regular basis.

A connection between high sugar intake and coronary artery disease was discovered in 1964. Research in 1993 revealed that alteration in carbohydrate metabolism is a significant risk factor for the development of cardiovascular disease. This is especially true for women who take birth control pills or hormones.

Impaired glucose tolerance is also described as one of the strongest predictors of adult-onset (noninsulin-dependent) diabetes. With insulin-dependent diabetes, positive actions to manage sugar and starch intake can help protect against associated secondary problems, such as neuropathy and blindness.

Digestive problems and chronic indigestion can result from excessive intake of sweets. *Candida albicans* and other microorganisms love sweet, simple, sugary foods. A sweet diet encourages greater infestation of bacteria, yeasts, and parasites, and will support their growth. Microbe infestation can also weaken our immunity. In addition, the presence of candida and other unfriendly organisms in our gut or other organ systems increases our craving for sweets, creating and perpetuating a negative cycle.

Frequent cravings for sweets can also be related to hypoglycemia (low blood sugar). Chronic low blood sugar can be the result of poor adrenal and pancreas function. However, we all get low blood sugar from time to time, when we skip a meal or work extra hard. If our blood sugar is low, a candy bar, a piece of cake, or an alcoholic beverage furnishes a quick "pick me up," reducing the symptoms of shakiness, fatigue, or anxiety. However, this relief is only short term. Sugar is absorbed so rapidly into the blood that the pancreas over-reacts to balance the glucose level. This can cause a rapid drop in blood sugar, which may result in mood swings with depression or anger. Orthomolecular medicine has suggested that some alcoholism may result from such hypoglycemic mood swings. In such cases, continuing to drink keeps the blood sugar up and the anxiety level down, but with negative long-term effects.

Sugar cravings are experienced commonly by women premenstrually, and chocolate is a common first choice. In Oriental medicine, the regular use or overuse of sugar is thought to lead to menstrual irregularities and premenstrual problems.

Sugar excess may also cause our bodies to age more rapidly. In 1993, geriatric researchers found that high calorie intake is a significant dietary factor responsible for aging. Empty calories from sweeteners and sweet foods may give us quick energy, but they also increase our energy utilization that stresses and ages our bodies more rapidly.

Our teeth are also subject to the destructive effects of sugar. When refined sugar was introduced into the diets of native peoples such as the Eskimos, New Zealand Maoris, and Australian aborigines, the number of dental cavities increased dramatically. In Europe and Japan, when sugar was rationed during World War II, the rate of cavities fell significantly. Research consistently shows that sugar and sticky starches destroy dental enamel and cause plaque and decay. Sweetened beverages are also linked to increased cavities. A major U.S. survey found that the use of soft drinks or sweet juices three or more times per day between meals doubled the chances of developing cavities.

CASE STUDY: JOHN B
Student and Restaurant Worker, age 22

I was 20 when I first met Dr. Haas. I was finishing up school and working part time, having just moved out from my folks' home. I wasn't doing very well. My emotions were all over the place; I was up and down, anxious and fatigued, and getting more run down. My checkup came out fine, and my folks encouraged me to see a psychiatrist. He put me on a couple of medications for depression, and then later a third and fourth one for my anxiety and poor sleep. I went back to see Dr. Haas a couple of months later. He was concerned about what I was doing. He had asked me to write down my diet for a few days, but I didn't do that (I guess I just couldn't face it).

On interviewing me, it came to light that I was addicted to Coca-Cola, Classic Coke to be exact, and I was drinking daily between one and two of what I remember was the 44-ounce size, the giant plastic bottles. The good doctor was quite alarmed. "Do you know the amount of sugar and caffeine you are consuming," he asked. Since I didn't, he showed me on paper. I was alarmed as well. He told me, "I am willing to bet you that if we can get off this cola habit, in a short time you won't need any of those medications, and after a week or two of transition, your moods and energy will feel more balanced. Then, your psychiatrist can start tapering you off of your medicines."

Well, that was a couple of years ago. And you know, Dr. Haas was mostly right. I am primarily off meds, yet I do have a tendency to depression and poor sleep. Yet, now I believe that if I am more diligent with my diet and take some supplements, these tendencies can be handled. However, I am still young and it's not always easy to be disciplined. Yet, I am grateful to Dr. Haas. He at least showed me that there are other ways to look at things, like health, and that non-drug solutions can really work. I am looking at a career in the health-care field because it seems a good way to help others.

Sugar and Its Effects on Children

Lifetime dietary habits are formed in infancy, so limiting the intake of sweets is of major importance. Blood sugar during infancy is less stable than later in childhood; thus babies are more susceptible to foods that rapidly raise and lower blood sugar. In fact, infant failure-to-thrive syndrome has been correlated with impaired carbohydrate metabolism, and specifically sucrose malabsorption. Some babies and young children develop chronic colic, cramping, and diarrhea from eating sugar, and this has been reported in the medical literature for more than twenty years.

Learning problems, exaggerated hyperactivity, and moodiness in children have all been linked to a high-sugar diet. Psychologists have observed decreased performance and increased inappropriate behavior following sugar intake. For certain children with attention-deficit hyperactivity disorder (ADHD), these effects can be more extreme. Not surprisingly, researchers found that decreasing sugar decreased socially inappropriate behavior.

The long-term effects of a sweet diet may actually be more severe than the immediate concerns. The habits we establish when we are young set the stage for lifetime patterns. A diet of empty calories may be a factor in frequent infections and failure to thrive. Extensive childhood dental cavities may result in teeth damaged beyond repair as an adult. Hypoglycemia in youth may result in recurring depression or alcoholism later in life. Chronic candida (yeast) infections, resulting from the frequent intake of sweets and the use of antibiotics, may set the stage for a lifetime of digestive and energy problems. Overweight children may become overweight adults, with the attendant increased risks for diabetes, cancer, and heart disease.

Decreasing the Sugar in Our Diet

Our intake of sweets is increasing, especially with the use of hidden sweeteners.

A quick look at the yearly statistics gives the impression that we are eating fewer sweets, because our sugar consumption has dropped from about 100 pounds a person to 64. Sounds good. However, our yearly intake of corn sweeteners has gone from about 20 pounds a person to more than 80. Our total intake of sweeteners is now about 150 pounds a year per person—almost a half pound of sweets per day.

Reducing sweeteners in our diet is a very real, positive step each of us can take. It requires an effort, but reducing our dietary load of sugar and sweeteners is of key importance for our health and our children's health.

The main artificial sweetener, aspartame (Nutrasweet), is not a worthy replacement. This substance is a neurological irritant and can affect a user's mood and energy. I have seen many people who do not tolerate this non-sugar sweetener similar to the way people do not tolerate MSG (monosodium glutamate, the flavor enhancer used commonly in Chinese cooking).

Sorbitol may be better tolerated and safer. However, the alcohol sweeteners such as sorbitol and mannitol are not well absorbed by the intestines, so they may cause gas and loose stools. Stevia is a natural alternative sweetener that is now widely available. It is an herb that most diabetics can use without risk of raising blood sugar levels. There are no known side effects, and it appears to be safe.

SUGAR SUBSTANCES ADDED TO FOODS

sucrose	fructose	dextrose
honey	malt syrup	maple sugar
corn syrup	high-fructose corn syrup	artificial sweetener

AVOID SUGAR FOODS AND SNACKS

WHITE SUGAR	CANDY	CAKE
soda pop	artificial juices	sweetened drinks
pies	puddings	cookies
ice cream	doughnuts	breakfast cereals
jello	corn syrup	liqueurs
jams & jellies	chewing gum	mixed drinks

AVOID HIDDEN SUGAR IN FOODS

BAKING MIXES	BREADS	CRACKERS
ketchup	relish	tartar sauce
salad dressings	cheese dips	soups
pickles	peanut butter	frankfurters
luncheon meats	prepared seafood	sausage
canned fruits	frozen vegetables	sweetened yogurt

The Glycemic Index

The Glycemic Index is a relatively new concept that relates to how quickly any sugars in foods are absorbed into the blood stream from the digestive tract. Basically, all simple sugars absorb quickly by themselves, with alcohol (a type of sugar) being absorbed quite rapidly. High glycemic foods are absorbed quickly, and lower glycemic foods, like oatmeal, are absorbed less quickly. Review the list on the next page, and you may be a bit surprised at what foods are high or low on the glycemic chart. If you eat foods lower on the glycemic index, your blood sugar will be more stable. When your blood sugar level is stable you will feel more energetic and likely experience less fatigue as well as less frequent mood shifts. Although we may strive to eat foods that are glycemically low, most of us end up eating some of the foods that are higher on the glycemic index now and then. Just be sure to eat them with high-fiber, slower absorbing starches or, more important, some protein food. For example, if you eat rice cakes, which are relatively high on the glycemic index, be sure to add nut butter (peanut butter, almond butter, cashew butter, and so forth), albacore tuna, or avocado slices, which are glycemically lower to help the rice cakes digest more slowly.

Low-carbohydrate diets are quite popular for weight loss these days, but there is a concern with excessive protein (and fats in some). Yet, there are healthy carbs (the complex starches and the high-fiber whole grains) and the fattening ones (the sugars and refined flour products). I suggest a diet with a good balance of wholesome foods that include fruits and whole grains along with lots of vegetables, some nuts and seeds, and individually needed proteins.

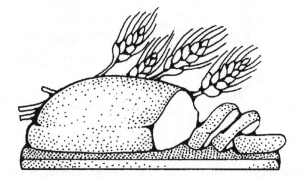

GLYCEMIC INDEX* OF CARBOHYDRATE FOODS

Note: Eating low on the index makes everything a little easier

Check out the Glycemic Index. Any food below fifty-five tends to conserve insulin and hormones. Overeating usually isn't a problem. It's the blast of insulin from foods high on the index that drives hunger cravings. With a diet of whole foods, appetite seems to drop quite naturally.

Grains, Breads, and Cereals

White bread	95
Instant rice	90
Rice cakes	80
Pretzels	80
Corn flakes	75
White flour	75
Graham crackers	75
Regular crackers	75
White bagel	75
Cheerios®	75
Puffed wheat	75
White rice	70
Taco shells	70
Spaghetti	60
Pita bread	55
Wild rice / brown rice	55
Oatmeal	55
Popcorn	55
Nuts	15–30

Fruits

Watermelon	70
Pineapple	65
Raisins	65–95
Ripe bananas	60
Mango, kiwi, grapes	50
Pears	45
Peaches, plums	40
Apples, oranges	40
Dried apricots	30–70
Grapefruit	25
Cherries	25

Vegetables

Baked potato	95
Parsnips	95
Carrots	85
French fries	80
Corn (sweet)	75
Beets	70
Sweet potatoes	55
Yams	50
Green peas	45
Green beans	45
Pinto beans	40
Lima beans	40
Butter beans	30
Black beans	30
Kidney beans	30
Artichoke	25
Asparagus	20
Tomatoes	15
Green vegetables	15

Dairy Products

Ice cream, premium	60
Yogurt, with fruit	35
Milk, whole	30+
Milk, skimmed	30
Yogurt, plain, no sugar	15

Sweeteners

Maltose	105–150
Glucose	100
Honey	75
Refined sugar	75

* Adapted from several sources, including *30-40-40: Fat-Burning Nutrition* by Daoust and *Sugar Busters* by Dr. Steward, et al.

Sugar Detox

Although sugar addiction is common, sugar withdrawal is usually physically mild, with periodic strong cravings. Emotional attachments and withdrawals may be more pronounced. For those who are sensitive to refined sugar or sweeteners, or who consume them in large amounts, genuine symptoms of abuse and withdrawal may occur. Some of these symptoms include fatigue, anxiety and irritability, depression and detachment, rapid heart rate and palpitations, and poor sleep. Most symptoms, if they do occur, last only a few days.

We can decide to cut down on or eliminate sugar quite easily by simply avoiding many of the sweet foods. There are plenty of nutritious nibbles to replace sugary snacks or treats—see below for suggestions. We should clear our cupboards of unhealthy sweetened foods. Once sugar has been removed from the diet, it is still possible to use it once in awhile, as it is not as re-addicting as many stronger drugs. Most people who have kicked the sugar habit find that they no longer tolerate sugar very well.

GOOD FOODS TO REPLACE SUGAR TREATS

fruit	vegetable sticks	granola
dried mango	salads	yogurt*
popcorn	almonds	peanuts
raisins	almond butter	peanut butter
mixed nuts	sunflower seeds	protein smoothies
edamame	pumpkin seeds	muesli

* Plain yogurt without the sweeteners is a healthful snack. Fresh fruit can be added along with seasonings such as vanilla, cinnamon, or nutmeg.

A diet that is rich in whole grains and other complex carbohydrates, vegetables, and protein foods can also help stabilize blood sugar and minimize the desire for sugar. Many people who are protein-deficient seem to crave sugars and carbohydrate foods. Conversely, eating a diet that focuses on protein and vegetables is a good way to minimize sugar cravings. If you don't tolerate sugars and sweet foods well, fruits should also be minimized and fruit juice avoided.

CASE STUDY: JEFF'S STORY
(age 52)

On our way to be Earth Guardian assistants for the last and most easterly stand of redwoods in Redwood Valley, California, we were joined by the realtor and her brother. During our journey, the tragic tale of her brother Jeff and his family was shared with us.

Two months prior, his wife of many years and the mother of his child committed suicide. Jeff moved in with his sister and spent his days lying on the couch with zero motivation. Of course, he had suffered a devastating loss.

His sister shared her observations. She saw her brother consuming over a six-pack of diet soda daily, including having a can at his bedside in a cooler at all times, which he drank throughout the night. She said, "Jeff, it's pretty clear you're not doing very well. Do you ever drink water or juice or anything else?" Jeff replied "Not really."

Now here's the story that he relayed. Two years prior, he and his wife realized that they had gained a little too much weight. They began a diet and included diet sodas to replace their use of sugar. They also added packets of the sweetener aspartame to other foods and beverages. Over the next few months, their moods began to shift and they became more and more depressed. They consulted a doctor who prescribed antidepressants for both of them. Without significant results, two other medicines were added over the next few months. None of their physicians interviewed them about their lifestyle habits.

As their moods and emotions became worse, one day Jeff came home and found a note next to the body of his wife who had shot and killed herself. "I can't go on, please care for our daughter." With this crisis, the daughter stayed with other relatives, and Jeff came to stay with his sister.

In response to the question about his diet soda use, they agreed to try an experiment. He shifted to drinking water and juice for several days. On the third day, he got off the couch and began washing and cleaning his car. Each day he began to feel better, and his mood became more positive. He was tapered off his medication and is now medicine- and diet soda-free and is actively participating in life. He believes, as I do, that he was having a reaction to the aspartame that affected his mood and nervous system. This is not uncommon.

This experience has inspired me to write a new book about the health-care system and how doctors can be more attentive to finding the real causes of most health problems.

As practitioners, if we do not explore with our patients their lifestyle choices and what effect each of them has on their energy, moods, and relationships, we cannot begin to address these important issues. If we only treat end results with medicines, and not address the underlying causes, then we are not practicing to the best of our capabilities.

We can clearly do better, and that is what my books and lifeworks are dedicated to—educating both patients and health-care practitioners to address and correct the true causes of illness and eliminating them.

And, by the way, the Redwood Forest was saved by an angel.

Supplements and Sugar

Nutrients that can help reduce the sugar craving and the symptoms of sugar withdrawal are the B vitamins, vitamin C, zinc, the trace mineral chromium, and the amino acid L-glutamine. Chromium is the central molecule of glucose, which helps insulin work more efficiently in removing sugar from the blood and nourishing the cells. L-glutamine, which can be used directly by the brain, is also helpful in reducing sugar (and alcohol) cravings.

Children can also benefit from a nutritional supplement program that includes some of the above mentioned nutrients, of course in lower dosages than for adults. Use of a good quality children's multi-vitamin/mineral, additional B vitamins to support the nervous system and general development, vitamin C at about 250 mg twice daily, and extra chromium (50 to 100 mcg 1 to 2 times daily) all help to minimize sugar cravings and to transition from sugar and sweetened foods. The supplement plan applies to children ages six to eleven; amounts may vary depending on the age and size of each child. These vitamins are water soluble and basically nontoxic. **However, if your child has a special problem or is below the age of six, you should check with your pediatrician or health-care provider for specific recommendations.**

The use of sugar in our culture resembles use of a drug and can be treated as such. Make a clear plan for withdrawal while working emotionally to eliminate the habit. Responses to flavors, certain food compulsions, and the feelings we get from them are usually conditioned. Self-reflection can be valuable. To change our habits, to stop and see things clearly, or to talk them through helps us transition from compulsion to the safe and balanced use of foods, sugar, and sweetened foods, as well as other substances we may use in our life.

"Heal your mother connection to your birth mother and your earth mother . . ."

—Bethany Argisle

OVERCOMING A SWEET TOOTH

1. Take sugar overconsumption seriously—it can have insidious negative effects over time. This is particularly true for young people later in their lives.

2. Eat a diet that includes vegetables, whole grains (complex carbohydrates), and protein. Increasing protein levels in the diet, both animal and vegetable, helps to reduce sugar cravings and use.

3. If you seriously overuse sugar, omit it (at least take a break to better understand your relationship to sugar) and consciously limit your intake of "hidden sweeteners" (particularly refined sugar [sucrose], corn syrup, and dextrose), and limit your use of honey and maple syrup. Eat some fruit, if you tolerate it, for natural sugar.

4. Support your body with extra helpful nutrients—these include the B vitamins, vitamin C, chromium, calcium, magnesium, and the amino acid L-glutamine.

5. Drink 8 glasses of water or herb tea a day.

6. Get sufficient fiber to keep your body cleansed and light.

7. If you suspect that you are hypoglycemic or diabetic, request the appropriate tests—such as a fasting blood sugar or a 5- or 6-hour glucose tolerance test—from your health-care practitioner.

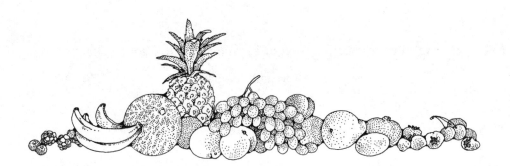

SUGAR DETOXIFICATION NUTRIENT PROGRAM

	ADULTS	CHILDREN
Water	2–3 qt	1–2 qt
Fiber	20–40 g	10–20 g
Vitamin E	200–800 IU	50–100 IU
Thiamine (B_1)	25–100 mg	10–50 mg
Riboflavin (B_2)	25–100 mg	10–25 mg
Niacinamide (B_3)	50–100 mg	10–50 mg
Pantothenic acid (B_5)	250–1,000 mg	50–250 mg
Pyridoxine (B_6)	25–100 mg	10–25 mg
Cobalamin (B_{12})	100–250 mcg	25–100 mcg
Folic acid	400–800 mcg	200–400 mcg
Vitamin C	2–10 g	500–1,000 mg
Bioflavonoids	250–500 mg	100–250 mg
Calcium	650–1,200 mg	350–600 mg
Chromium	200–500 mcg	100–250 mcg
Magnesium	400–800 mg	200–400 mg
Manganese	5–10 mg	3–5 mg
Selenium	200–300 mcg	50–100 mcg
Vanadium	200–400 mcg	50–100 mcg
Zinc	30–60 mg	15–30 mg
L-amino acids	1,000–1,500 mg	250–500 mg
L-glutamine	500–1,000 mg	0
Essential fatty acids	2–4 capsules	0
or Flaxseed oil	2–4 teaspoons	1–2 capsules
Adrenal glandular	100–200 mg	0

I believe sugar is the number one addiction on our planet. Take a break some time and see how you feel. You may feel more real.

CHAPTER EIGHT

Nicotine Detoxification

◆

The cigarette is the world's most profitable globally distributed product. Why? Because nicotine is more addictive than either alcohol or cocaine. However, in recent years the U.S. courts and people have made the cigarette companies pay big money back to the smokers (and their lawyers and the health-care system) who have been injured from their addiction. Nicotine pushers didn't tell the public that smoking was so addictive, and they still downplay this fact and appear to have little concern about getting new customers hooked on their product.

Cigarette smoking, our primary method of using nicotine, is the single greatest cause of preventable disease and probably creates the most difficult addiction to deal with. The statistics are shocking: Worldwide, 2.5 million people per year die of tobacco-related diseases. In the United States alone, cigarette smoking causes over 1,000 deaths per day and is responsible for about 25 percent of cancer deaths and 30 to 40 percent of coronary heart disease deaths.

Cigarette smoking also increases the incidence of atherosclerosis, strokes, and peripheral vascular disease. Diseases of the respiratory tract—colds, flus, acute bronchitis, pneumonia, chronic obstructive pulmonary diseases (COPD) such as emphysema and chronic bronchitis, and lung cancer—are all much more common in smokers. Infections and allergies are also prevalent in smokers, as is rapid aging of the body, especially facial skin, which results from the poor oxygenation of tissues and other associated chemical effects.

Smoking clearly decreases life expectancy for all age groups. One-pack-a-day smokers double their chance of death between ages fifty and sixty, while two-packers triple theirs. (These statistics are reflected in the insurance rates smokers pay, which are twice that of non-smokers.) Smoking also affects the life expectancy of family non-smokers. Of all the commonly used drugs, nicotine has the least benefits and the greatest consequences.

Despite these facts, some 650 billion cigarettes are sold yearly in the United States, creating an $18 to $25 billion megabusiness. The 650 billion count averages to about 4,000 cigarettes per year per person over the age of eighteen, although aggressive marketing and social pressure targets people even younger. The total cost of caring for people with health problems caused by cigarette smoking is staggering at about $72.7 billion per year, according to health economists at the University of California.

The 1989 Surgeon General's Report stated that about half of all smokers begin before the age of fifteen. Recent estimates suggest that about 38 percent of the over-eighteen population in the United States smoke. Nearly all women who smoke started as teenagers, while 30 percent of high school senior girls are still current smokers. Percentages of adult smokers are much higher in most European countries and parts of Asia. Billions of dollars are spent to treat the problems that afflict smokers, and many more billions are lost due to decreased work and productivity.

Children getting hooked on cigarettes is the saddest part of the nicotine story. We must insist on more stringent laws to better regulate sales and advertising, along with better education to help curtail this problem.

Since most nicotine is ingested by smoking cigarettes, that is the focus of this chapter. Cigar and pipe smoking, chewing tobacco and snuff also pose health risks, but far fewer than with cigarettes. Tobacco comes from a large-leafed nightshade, or *Solanaceae,* plant. It is one of only a few plants that contain the psychoactive alkaloid nicotine. Tobacco causes joint pain in some people, which correlates with the theory that arthritis is in part due to a nightshade allergy.

The highly addictive nature of nicotine is revealed by the fact that many strong-minded and strong-willed people cannot stop smoking, even if they are otherwise health conscious. Over 80 percent of smokers say that they want to stop. In my years working in hospitals, I saw lung cancer and emphysema patients smoking between ventilator treatments and patients with tubes in their necks from tracheostomies putting cigarettes into the tubes to inhale.

NICOTINE EFFECTS AND BENEFITS (YES, THERE ARE A FEW)

Many people find smoking to be relaxing, but this may be related to the way it calms hyperactive withdrawal symptoms. People do experience increased mental stimulation and improved hand-to-eye coordination as a result of nicotine's vascular-neurological stimulation, but the effects do not last.

The "up" feeling that smoking produces is probably correlated with increased blood pressure and heart rate, as well as the production of fatty acids, steroids, hormones, and neurotransmitters (and also from easing the withdrawal). Nicotine mimics acetylcholine, which improves alertness, memory, and learning capacity. Stimulation of norepinephrine and endorphins by nicotine may help balance moods and increase energy. The liver's increased glycogen release gives a satisfying lift to the blood sugar.

Dr. Tom Ferguson's book *The Smoker's Book of Health* cites how hundreds of smokers said they felt better able to deal with stress and to relax with nicotine. Smoking helped control their moods, improved concentration and energy levels (especially with fatigue), and reduced withdrawal symptoms. Social comfort, work breaks, reduced pain and anxiety, increased pleasure, and less boredom were also noted.

Smoking also reduces one's appetite and taste for food, a benefit for the weight conscious. In fact, the average smoker weighs six to eight pounds less than the non-smoker. In the book *Life Extension* (out of print), Sandy Shaw and Durk Pearson note that nicotine seems to reduce distraction by outside stimuli in people working in highly stimulating environments—that is, it desensitizes people.

Nicotine is a mild central nervous system stimulant and a strong cardiovascular system stimulant. It constricts blood vessels, increasing blood pressure and stimulating the heart, and raises blood fat levels. In its liquid form, nicotine is a powerful poison— the injection of even one drop would be deadly. Interestingly, it is the nicotine, not the smoke, that causes people to continue smoking cigarettes, yet it is the smoking itself that causes so many of the health problems.

The initial irritating effects of nicotine easily progress to chronic irritations, yet these are outweighed by the physiological and psychological dependence. People addicted to heroine and other powerful drugs have commonly cited nicotine as the hardest drug to kick. The American Psychiatric Association has described smoking as an "organic mental disorder." Their statistics suggest that around 50 percent of people cannot stop smoking when they try to and that of the people who do stop, about 75 percent of them begin again within one year.

Cigarette smoke is a combination of lethal gases (carbon monoxide, hydrogen cyanide, and nitrogen and sulfur oxides) and tars (which contain an estimated four thousand chemicals). Some of these chemical agents are introduced by the actual manufacturing processes. Tobacco has been smoked for centuries, and it has until recently been naturally grown and dried. It appears that in the last century, as chemicals have been added, the negative effects of smoking have skyrocketed. Research suggests that natural tobacco poses much less cancer and cardiovascular disease risk than processed tobacco.

WHAT ARE THE RISKS OF SMOKING?

Dangers in modern tobacco products include pesticides used during cultivation and chemicals added to the tobacco to make it burn better or taste different. Chemicals added to the leaves and papers to enhance burning are the major cause of fire death in this country, as those cigarettes continue to burn after they have been put down. Forced burning also makes people smoke more of each cigarette in order to keep up with it. Sugar curing and rapid flue drying are also associated with increased toxicity. Kerosene heat drying contaminates the tobacco with yet another toxic hydrocarbon. If a cigarette does not go out when left alone, it has been chemically treated. Using a natural tobacco may reduce smoking risks.

Other toxic contaminants in cigarettes include cadmium (which affects the kidneys, arteries, and blood pressure), lead, arsenic, cyanide, and nickel. Dioxin, the most toxic pesticide chemical known, has been found in cigarettes, as has acetonitrile, another pesticide. The nitrogen gases from cigarettes generate carcinogenic nitrosamines in body tissues. The tars in smoke contain polynuclear aromatic hydrocarbons (PAHs), carcinogenic materials that bind with cellular DNA to cause damage. Antioxidant therapy, particularly with vitamin C, helps protect against both PAH and nitrosamines. Extra C blocks the irritating effects of smoke and replaces what is lost due to reduced absorption (blood levels of ascorbic acid average about 30 to 40 percent lower in smokers than in nonsmokers).

Radioactive materials are also found in cigarette smoke, polonium being the most common. Some authorities believe that cigarettes are our greatest source of radiation, which is a strong aging factor. A smoker of one and a half packs per day may be exposed to radiation levels equal to three hundred chest X rays yearly. Acetaldehyde, a chemical released during smoking, also causes aging (especially of the skin) as it affects the cross-linking bonds that hold our tissues together.

There are different levels of nicotine addiction. Least addicted are those who smoke socially—only at parties with friends—and usually only during certain times of the day or week. Next are those who smoke in response to stress, mainly at work, and who may stop and start periodically. These two types usually find it easier to cut down or stop. Those of us who are all-day-long smokers have a strong physical and psychological addiction. Going more than an hour without nicotine brings on withdrawal symptoms such as irritability, anxiety, or headache. Often, the psychological factors are more intense than the physical ones. Consuming two or more packs a day indicates a strong addiction; medical and psychological support will likely be necessary to quit successfully. Specialized smoking-cessation programs are often useful.

Contrary to current marketing hype about low-tar, low-nicotine cigarettes, there are no safe smoking options. Some of the newer "lights" may be even worse than regular cigarettes as users inhale more deeply and smoke more frequently in order to satisfy nicotine needs. More carbon monoxide, hydrogen cyanide, and nitrogen gases are consumed with many of these low-nicotine cigarettes, and this can increase the oxygen deficit, heart disease, and lung damage associated with smoking.

What smokers really need are high-nicotine, low-tar cigarettes, so that they will smoke less for the same amount of nicotine (this is what a nicotine patch does, for example). Even better would be a way to get nicotine to the blood without smoke at all. Nicotine gum works well, and nicotine skin patches are now used in smoking-cessation programs. Nicotine nasal sprays have just been released, and soon there may be capsules or tablets to satisfy the craving.

PROBLEMS ASSOCIATED WITH SMOKING

Cough	Allergies	Cancers
Hoarseness	Rhinitis/sinusitis	Lung
Headaches	Lowered immunity	Mouth and tongue
Anxiety	Other infections	Larynx
Fatigue	Blood disorders	Esophagus
Leg pains	Nutrient deficiencies	Bladder
Cold hands and feet	Acute bronchitis	Cervix
Memory loss	Chronic bronchitis	Pancreas
Senility	Emphysema	Kidney
Alzheimer's disease	Increased cholesterol	Surgical complications
Rapid skin aging	Atherosclerosis	Increased pregnancy risks
Teeth and finger stains	Hypertension	Increased infant mortality
Periodontal disease	Angina pectoris	Burns from fires
Low libido	Circulation insufficiency	Increased caffeine use
Impotence	Heart and artery disease	Increased alcohol use
Heartburn	Heart attacks and strokes	More job and home changes
Peptic ulcers	Varicose veins	Higher insurance and
Hiatal hernia	Osteoporosis	medical fees

All of these options will still be moderately hazardous to our health, but much less so than smoking. They will also get rid of the primary and secondary risks due to smoke and smoke-borne chemicals.

Although about a third of adult men and women in the United States smoke, over one million of the over fifty million smokers in the United States stop smoking each year; when we do this, we immediately begin to lower our potential for disease.

Cigarette smoking puts us at risk through three primary degenerative-disease producing effects: 1) irritation and inflammation; 2) free-radical generation; and 3) allergy-addiction. Respiratory and cardiovascular diseases are the greatest and deadliest long-term consequences of smoking.

- **Cardiovascular disease** (CVD), or the process of artherosclerosis, from the inflammatory effects and cholesterol-increasing effects of nicotine on the circulatory system.

- **CVD** from carbon monoxide in inhaled smoke, which reduces the delivery of oxygen to our cells.

- **Reduced oxygen** levels cause our body to produce more red blood cells (polycythemia).

- **CVD** is primarily responsible for the **decreased life expectancy** associated with smoking, even more so than with lung cancer, which usually only arises after 20 to 30 years of use, while circulatory effects start immediately.

- The three primary contributors to CVD are **smoking, hypertension,** and **high cholesterol,** and smoking increases the incidence of the latter two.

- Nicotine also lowers the level of the protective HDL cholesterol.

- Decreased circulation and increased peripheral vascular resistance cause the heart to work harder with every beat and contributes to **elevated blood pressure.**

- Increased platelet aggregation leads to **strokes** and **heart attacks.** Smokers are three times more likely than nonsmokers to suffer heart attacks, mostly of the artery-spasm type. The pre-heart attack propensity to angina pectoris is also higher. Nicotine (and other agents in smoke) increases the incidence of **arrhythmias** (irregular heartbeat).

- **Cerebral aneurysm** (ballooning of the artery wall) may also be fatal.

- **Peripheral vascular disease** (disease of the arteries in the extremities) may manifest as **intermittent claudication** (pain in the legs when walking), as the poor circulation caused by atherosclerosis and vasoconstriction reduces oxygen delivery to the muscles.

- **Buerger's disease** is an arterial disease that may be caused by a hypersensitivity or allergy to tobacco. The inflammation and scarring of the arteries in the arms and legs may even lead to amputation.

- Chronic inhalation of tobacco smoke eventually **destroys lung tissue** through a process of irritation, inflammation, and scarring.

- A higher than average incidence of **respiratory infections**, including **colds and flus**, bronchitis and sinusitis. Cigarette smoke causes temporary paralysis of the cilia (fine hairs on the mucous linings that protect the deeper tissues from microorganisms and other foreign materials). The thinning and drying of the mucus itself dries and irritates the bronchial tubes.

- **Chronic bronchitis,** one form of **chronic obstructive pulmonary disease (COPD)**, results from long-term irritation, loss of mucus protection, and recurrent infection with a subsequent **loss of lung capacity and function.** This limitation in respiratory function occurs very near the onset of smoking. When smoking is stopped, much of the function returns, unless there is lung tissue scarring, which is irreversible.

- Smoking generally decreases lung capacity and endurance and with it, the desire or ability to exercise. **Emphysema,** another form of COPD, results from progressive scarring and loss of lung elasticity.

- Smokers are five to ten times more likely to contract **lung cancer** than nonsmokers. These rates are even further increased with occupational exposure to agents such as asbestos, coal, textiles, and other chemicals. With regular alcohol use, smokers have greater than fifteen times the risk of lung cancer than nonsmokers.

- Many other cancer rates are also higher for smokers, particularly for alcohol-drinking smokers who are exposed to other **carcinogenic chemicals.**

- **Allergy-addiction** symptoms may appear when smoking is first begun and then decrease with continued smoking.

- Increased **atherosclerosis** and subsequent decrease in blood circulation to the brain lead to **memory loss** and thinking problems, as well as early dementia. Recent research shows that smokers have twice the risk of **Alzheimer's disease.**

- Poor oxygen delivery to the skin and general dehydration of the tissues caused by smoking **ages the skin** and increases the number of deep wrinkles.

- Worldwide reports show how smoking affects **sexuality and reproduction.** In men, smoking has been shown to **lower sperm counts** and reproductive ability. Smoking may also cause genetic mutation, as there appears to be a slightly higher incidence of congenital malformations in the offspring of men who smoke.

- In women who smoke, there are clearly more **miscarriages** and babies with lower birth weights.

- Smoking also increases the incidence of **stillbirths, congenital malformations,** and **early infant deaths.**

- Smoking around newborns and infants increases their susceptibility to many diseases, particularly **colds, ear infections, bronchitis, and pneumonia.**

- Women are at risk for all of the problems described in this list, but are particularly vulnerable if they are using birth control pills. For example, women who smoke and use the pill are 25 times more likely to suffer a heart attack than women who do neither.

- Although **snuff** and **chewing tobacco** are less toxic, chronic use of nicotine affects the circulatory system. There are currently over 10 million chewers addicted to nicotine; even though they are not exposed to smoke, they still have the negative cardiovascular effects and a higher incidence of mouth, tongue, and throat cancers than smokers. The smoke from cigars and pipes is not usually inhaled (some is), so less nicotine and tars are absorbed with their use, although local irritation is possible.

- Smoking reduces appetite and taste for food, thus **interfering with good nutrition.**

- Increased risk of **osteoporosis** due to poor calcium utilization.

- Increased incidence of **heartburn, hiatal hernia,** and **peptic ulcers.**

- Increased **risk of fire.**

HIGH-RISK SMOKERS

Pregnant women	Obese people
Nursing mothers	Very thin people
Diabetics	Alcoholics or alcohol abusers (daily users)
Women using birth control pills	People with existing smoker's disease
People with family history of heart disease	People who work with toxic chemicals
People with high blood pressure	People having surgery
People with high cholesterol	Ulcer patients
Heavy smokers	Type A personalities

SMOKING

by Bethany Argisle

Smoking grew from an experiment into a way of life, a habit, and ulti-mately, a relationship. And as the pressure of my existence (now called stress) added up both for and against me, I found the perfect excuse/reason/alliance with my smoking relationship.

At the age of twenty, I fulfilled my destiny and got a job in the major metropolitan newspaper that I had in my sights, something I had always wanted. So many folks smoked during the 1960s—I openly became one of them—up to three packs a day. So what if I had more attacks of bronchitis, more phlegm, and colds. I got my work finished each day in a frenzy of deadlines, activities, and freeway driving. Through my career, lovers, marriage, and stresses of Los Angeles smog and mere money and family, I always returned to my primal fire desire, my cigarette.

My dad was the supervisor for United Artists Theatres, and the movies were big in my life. So many movie queens and sirens smoked. It made them tough and desirable, mystical almost; it made them have something of their own, the power of fire.

Men loved to buy me drinks (yes, a drink and a cigarette)…substance nirvana! There were newspaper bars where many real stories were told by the firelight of my nicotine torch. These were the days when we hacked in private and no one yet had announced lung cancer or the dec-imation and wasting of the lungs of the planet, the forests.

During my *Times* tenure, we launched ourselves into space and lost our resident president. All the while, I worked under the daily deadlines and socio stresses. Then I smoked for different reasons, I couldn't stop! I had to have it from morning to night and even though I always was hygienic, my clothes smelled and I doused myself and brushed to pretend to mask the effect. I had become a Vixen of Vapors, living my habit…

Now, I cringe at what I could have done with all that lung power, all that money and energy. After reading *Global Dreams* and observing several wealthy people go down from emphysema, I realized what I had done to my body machine I was given to live in. Yet, at that time I didn't know. Did I quit? Absolutely NOT!

There was no such thing as quitting, so I continued and no one said much except for my mother and her "coffin nails" speech. Years passed, and of course my lung capacity and therefore my brain and heart capacity diminished, but I was young and the stain of pain was not permanent, or so I thought.

Then, I couldn't take it anymore, I had an auto accident, almost caught my room on fire in the hospital by throwing a lighted cig in the trash under the "No Smoking" sign.

After my accident and news career, I serendipitously became a storyteller, even though I was being offered more mere money to continue my high-stress lifestyle. My accident became my guide for what made life better for my heart. One day after a very touching story session, I went into another room as the children were leaving. A little girl surprised me and came running up to me, all decked out in a hoop skirt and crown and went to hug me. Little did she know that I already had a lighted cigarette in my hand and was sucking in the chems and smoke to appease my fire Goddess. She grabbed my hand and was immediately burned. Instead of the joy she came to share, my habit collided with her innocent spirit.

This affected me greatly and after tending to her, I went home with my head and lungs hung in remorse. All night long I felt as if I were at a crossroads, a death of some sort. I felt shame for bringing pain to this dear innocent one. That night I decided I would not any longer, I just could not, smoke cigarettes again. No more smokestackin' for me.

All that freed up energy, I began to sing, to perform. I knew symbolically the little girl was the little girl in me. She was an answer to a prayer I didn't know I prayed and wherever she is, she is my angel...

You smokers, you tokers, I encourage you to face the discomfort, the failure, and improve the use and focus of your energy. I was the first person I knew who quit completely and believe me, it wasn't easy to see that others acted as I did when I was a prisoner of my habit. Of course, if you read Dr. Haas's first book *Staying Healthy with the Seasons,* you will learn that fire creates earth. People seek fire for stimulation to get things done. So, with some studying, I began to see/feel/know that I was addicted to one cycle. Now my challenge is staying healthy, not getting healthy.

What About Secondary Smoke?

Secondary smoke has become a human rights issue in the last decade as people feel that it is a violation of their right to breathe clean air. Secondhand smoke is potentially more dangerous than mainstream smoke because it is not filtered. Of the sixteen or so poisons that arise from burning cigarettes, most are known carcinogens. Much of the ammonia, formaldehyde, acetaldehyde, formic acid, phenol, hydrogen sulfide, acetonitrile, and methyl chloride is filtered through the cigarette filters and is more concentrated in the smoke that wafts into the air. This is the smoke that passive, involuntary smokers inhale. Carbon monoxide levels in secondhand smokers is more than 50 percent higher than that of those not exposed and often even exceeds that of light firsthand smokers.

A review of more than 2,000 studies regarding secondhand smoke suggests that it increases the incidence of most of the diseases associated with smoking. Children of smokers have increased incidence of respiratory infections, ear infections, and lower lung function than children of nonsmokers. Secondhand smoke increases the risk of COPD, heart disease, and lung cancer. In fact, an estimated three thousand cases of lung cancers per year are caused by secondhand smoking. It has been found that nonsmoking wives of male smokers have life expectancies that are four years shorter than those of nonsmoking wives of nonsmokers.

HOW DO WE DETOXIFY FROM NICOTINE?

A good air filter is an important preventive measure and can be very effective in removing toxins from the air; a basic multiple vitamin-mineral and antioxidant formula will help protect us internally. The daily program should include at least:

SMOKER'S SIMPLE NUTRIENT PLAN	
Vitamin C	1,000–2,000 mg, up to 6–8 grams daily
Mixed carotenoids*	15,000–25,000 IU, up to 50,000 IU
Vitamin A	5,000–10,000 IU
Zinc	15–30 mg
Selenium	200 mcg
Vitamin E	400 IU

* Note: Even though beta-carotene did not fare well in recent studies for smokers when used solely, I believe its action within a complete antioxidant formula is still warranted based on a number of other positive studies. Here, the mixed carotenoids are likely more helpful than beta-carotenes alone.

Dietary Recommendations

No support program for smokers will be as effective as ceasing to smoke completely and working to regain lost health. A wholesome diet and nutritional supplements can help protect us from some of the effects of smoking; however, even the best program cannot offer immunity. There is a tendency for poor dietary habits to accompany the destructive smoking habit. Many smokers tend to eat more meats, fatty, fried, and refined foods than nonsmokers, although there are smoking vegetarians, smoking exercise fanatics, and smoking health enthusiasts.

This plan, with adequate fruits, vegetables, and whole grains, will help to replenish the protective antioxidant nutrients such as vitamins C, E, and A, beta-carotene, and selenium. In addition, raw seeds and nuts, legumes, sprouts, and other proteins should be consumed. Water is essential to balance out the drying effects of smoking and its toxicity. Caffeine also increases the need for water, as it is dehydrating. A daily intake of two to three quarts of liquid is suggested, depending on how many high-water-content fruits, vegetables, salads, juices, and soups are consumed.

Since smoking usually generates an acidic condition in the body, I recommend following the New Detox Diet plan. A high-fiber diet helps detoxification by maintaining bowel function.

The nutritional strategy for smokers is to increase the intake of wholesome foods—fruits, vegetables, and whole grains—and to decrease the intake of fats and fried foods, cured or pickled products, food additives, and alcohol. The increased blood and tissue alkalinity that results from this diet helps reduce the craving for and interest in smoking, as shown by studies and my patients' reports.

An alkaline diet is not necesarily needed over an entire lifetime, although generally, it is preferable to an acidic diet. During cigarette withdrawal, a vegetarian or raw food diet may sufficiently reduce nicotine craving and can be used for three to six weeks to

---

STOP SMOKING DIET

Increase Alkaline Foods		Reduce Acid Foods	
Examples:		*Examples:*	
fruits	figs	meats	beef
vegetables	raisins	sugar	chicken
greens	carrots	wheat	eggs
lima beans	celery	bread	milk
millet	almonds	baked goods	cheese

aid in the detoxification process. Fasting has also been employed by some smokers to help eliminate their habit. It is a means of rapid transition, but is also somewhat intense. A juice fast under medical supervision might best be used with the very determined person or with the overweight or hypertensive smoker.

Several weeks of the Detox Diet (page 73) can be very effective at clearing the smoker's desire, habit, and chemicals from the body. Over a longer time, a vegetarian diet high in chlorophyllic (green) vegetables and sprouts, grains, fruits, and liquids such as water, juices, soups, and herbal teas is preferable. The raw foods diet is similar, but includes more seeds and nuts. Eating raw, unsalted sunflower seeds (or carrot or celery sticks) can help replace that hand-to-mouth habit we reinforce when we smoke. However, we must be careful not to replace nicotine addiction with new food addictions, but with better exercise and breathing habits, gardening, massage and so on.

The diet for detoxification is low in fat and high in fiber, helping to keep energy levels high and the gut cleansed. Raw and vegetarian foods help with both. The diet includes several salads of leafy greens daily, and some fruit, vegetable, nut, or seed snacks. Some of the high-protein algaes such as spirulina, blue-green algae, or chlorella also help during withdrawal and detox.

Supplements

To support body alkalinization during smoking cessation, take sodium or potassium bicarbonate tablets; take one to two during each period of craving up to a total of five or six tablets daily. A general "multiple" vitamin/mineral with additional antioxidant nutrients is an important part of the smoker's program (see page 141 for all dosages). The antioxidants help reduce the toxicity of smoke in primary and secondary smokers and also help lessen free-radical irritation during the detox period.

Vitamin E helps stabilize cell membranes, protecting them and the tissue membranes from free-radical and chemical irritations. Selenium, as sodium selenite or selenomethionine, supports vitamin E and also reduces cancer potential. Selenium also lessens sensitivity to cadmium. Vitamin A reduces cancer risk and supports tissue health; beta-carotene may still offer some protection against the problems of smoking when used with other antioxidants.

Smokers need regular vitamin C intake to help neutralize the toxins and compensate for reduced absorption. (Note: Since both vitamin C and niacin are mild acids, they may aggravate any irritations in the gut, and thus may increase ulcer risk as well as nicotine cravings in smokers. If C or niacin is used in higher amounts, added alkaline salts such as the bicarbonates or calcium-magnesium ascorbates may be used.)

Extra zinc, 30 to 60 mg a day, like vitamin A, helps protect the tissue and mucous membranes and reduces cadmium toxicity and absorption. If higher levels of zinc (over 60 mg daily) are taken, supplement with 3 to 4 mg copper and 5 to 10 mg of manganese.

We need the support of the B vitamins, particularly thiamine (B_1), pyridoxine (B_6), and cobalamin (B_{12}). B_{12} is thought to help decrease the cellular damage caused by tars and nicotine. Niacin (B_3) helps open up constricted circulation. It also lowers cholesterol, which may reduce the risk of atherosclerosis. Pantothenic acid (B_5) may reduce skin aging and the effects of stress. Folic acid should be taken in higher amounts, 1 to 2 mg or more, and offers some cardiovascular protection. Coenzyme Q10 can be helpful, and extra choline supports the brain and memory. Magnesium and molybdenum are also needed in higher amounts than usual.

L-cysteine (along with thiamine and vitamin C) protects the lungs from acetaldehyde generated by smoking, and helps reduce smoker's cough. This can be taken in the form of NAC (n-acetyl-cysteine) 250 mg two to three times daily. Glutathione, formed from L-cysteine, is part of the protective antioxidant enzyme system. Heavy smokers might use 250 to 500 mg of glutathione, up to 1,500 mg (usually 500 to 750 mg) of L-cysteine, with 5 to 6 g of vitamin C, 150 mg thiamine, and the total B vitamins and a balanced amino acid formula daily.

To prevent obesity during and following smoking cessation, it is very important to be aware of our eating habits. Since smoking reduces appetites and increases metabolism, it is natural to want to eat more when not smoking. Replace smoking with exercise or new activities. Research has shown that smokers crave and eat less sweets than nonsmokers; however, this changes with smoking cessation as the taste buds come alive again. Over half of ex-smokers will gain weight when they stop smoking, and this is even more common in the heavier-use smokers. If weight gain is undesirable (many smokers are underweight and should gain weight), a weight-control diet should be instituted as smoking is stopped. The alkaline, high-fiber, low-fat diet is helpful in maintaining weight. Another amino acid, L-phenylalanine, can help reduce the appetite if taken before meals in amounts of 250 to 500 mg. However, its mild tendency to raise blood pressure should be taken into consideration. (This may be countered by the tendency of the blood pressure to drop somewhat with smoking cessation.) More choline may improve fat utilization and maintain weight, as may the amino acid L-carnitine. Regular exercise and plenty of fresh air are also part of the plan.

The level of nicotine addiction is based upon daily amounts and total number of years smoking, and will determine the ease of cessation. If you light up first thing in the morning or if you smoke more than two packs a day, it may be harder for you to stop than for lighter smokers.

STOP-SMOKING PLANS

There are many different cessation plans. The best way is just to make a firm decision and go cold turkey—there is no back and forth, no doubt; the decision is made. The success rate for those who make this bold move is much better than for those who use other methods. They do not need tapes, counselors, or group support; they count on themselves. Those who depend on others to stop smoking have more relapses.

Withdrawal is not easy. The first three days to a week can be very difficult; for some people, the struggle may last for months. Usually, the first twelve to twenty-four hours are the peak of withdrawal, when symptoms may appear and when cigarette craving is almost omnipresent. During withdrawal, take one gram of vitamin C (as a mineral ascorbate—calcium or magnesium—to reduce acidity) every one or two hours. This may help reduce nicotine cravings.

If you just cannot give up nicotine, there are other ways to get rid of cigarettes. Though not ideal, they are at least one step better than smoking. Nicorette, a nicotine gum, is now available without prescription and can be a very useful transitional tool; nicotine patches in varying strengths are also being used.

If you won't give it up, and your mate or significant other won't, you have a challenge to face.

In a January 2003 article in *The Journal of Clinical Investigation,* the American Lung Association commented that a recent laboratory study suggested that nicotine used to help smokers quit may even promote lung cancer. However, The American Lung Association continues to endorse nicotine replacement therapy (NRT). Over 100 clinical trials (including a National Institutes of Health-supported study involving people who used nicotine gum for five years) and extensive use over a number of years have proven the safety and efficacy of NRT products when used as directed. In direct contrast, tobacco smoke contains over forty known carcinogens, plus many other toxins, such as carbon monoxide, arsenic, and ammonia as well as substances that can trigger heart disease, emphysema, and many other life-threatening diseases.

Leading experts in the field of smoking control agree that NRT products have a crucial role to play in helping to reduce the devastating toll of disease caused by tobacco dependence. The concern is, however, that people will abuse these patches and gum, using them while also smoking. We suggest only using NRTs as directed by the manufacturer. Call your local American Lung Association at 1-800-LUNG-USA (1-800-586-4872) to find out more about their ideas of how to stop smoking for good.

Both methods used commonly for smoking cessation, nicotine gum and patches, support nicotine addiction without harmful smoke chemicals. They reduce withdrawal symptoms, and research suggests a better long-term quitting percentage for those using. These are, however, temporary aids. These substances may cause nausea, light-headedness, hiccups, and muscle tension or jaw aches from chewing. They do, however, immediately help one to stop smoking, as most of the nicotine craving is satisfied. The smoking response must still be addressed, and the former smoker should be off the gum or patches within a couple of months, or sometimes longer. (Patches may even need to be used for a year to be successful.) Research suggests that people with ulcers or cardiovascular disease should avoid these methods, as should pregnant women. "Smokeless" cigarettes can be used for withdrawal and transition as well.

If none of these methods are successful for you, there are many self-help suggestions for cutting down. Working to smoke fewer cigarettes daily is a common practice, but generally ten per day is needed to satisfy the nicotine habit. You might also try taking fewer puffs per cigarette or smoking just the first half of each, where the least amounts of tars and chemicals are concentrated. Filters and cigarette holders decrease the amount of toxic elements inhaled. There are also devices that place tiny holes in cigarette filters to allow dilution of smoke with outside air. You might also try changing brands to lower-tar, higher-nicotine cigarettes or using brands you do not like. For anyone who smokes, avoid chemically treated cigarettes and using natural, untreated tobacco and untreated paper.

Compose a plan and schedule of cessation dates and stages of nonsmoking before quitting, and document your reasons for doing so. Pick a low-stress time to stop, such as during vacation or just after sick leave from work or school. New Year's Day, your birthday, or national stop smoking days are other good choices. Keep notes of your process and feelings. Get to know yourself better through this process; many smokers release a lot of energy and excitement as they quit, so use this to construct new and better habits in all areas of your life.

When you quit, make a commitment. If you have trouble doing this, find someone with lung cancer or emphysema to talk with. Know your cigarette triggers and work to defuse them. Get rid of ashtrays, clean your teeth and your home, and make your life a nonsmoking zone. Take extra special care of yourself with good foods, pure drinking water, hot baths or showers, exercise, and massage. Reward yourself with a trip to the mountains, an afternoon off at the movies, a day at a spa or beauty salon. Get your mind off yourself by getting involved with others: try volunteer work; coach or play on a softball team; organize a fund-raiser for your community. Learn a new language or musical instrument; try gardening or a new sport. Breathe fresh air, walk, and get your heart beating harder.

SUGGESTIONS FOR SMOKING CESSATION

- Cut down on other addictive substances, such as caffeine, sugar, and alcohol, all of which can increase the desire to smoke.

- Get another smoker to stop with you or, even better, get an ex-smoker to support you while you stop.

- Tell empathetic friends or family and ask for their support—that is, go public with your plan to stop.

- Stay busy to prevent boredom and to keep your mind off smoking.

- Exercise regularly to decrease withdrawal, increase motivation, and increase relaxation. Include your favorite aerobic sport and try to do it outdoors.

- If you are not an exerciser, consider taking yoga, swimming, or low-impact aerobics.

- Create rewards for being successful and implement them daily.

- Get plenty of rest.

- Drink fluids and use water for therapy by taking showers, baths, saunas, or hot tubs, or by going swimming.

- Change daily patterns to avoid stimulating old smoking conditioning. This may include staying away from bars, alcohol, and coffee, avoiding friends who smoke, not receiving or making phone calls at specific locations in which you usually smoked, and getting up and doing something right after a meal.

- Learn and practice relaxation and breathing techniques.

- Practice visualization.

- Keep a positive attitude toward health and life.

- Get health treatments, such as massage or teeth cleaning to remove cigarette stains.

- Find temporary oral substitutes to deal with psychological ties to smoking. Oral fixation substitutes could include munchies such as vegetable sticks (carrot, celery, zucchini), apples, nuts, popcorn, sunflower seeds (unsalted) in shells, sugarless hard candies or non-edible substitutes such as gum; or chewing or sucking on ice cubes, toothpicks, licorice sticks, or drinking straws.

- If cravings arise, find ways to deal with them: Take a short break, a walk, a shower, drink tea, or do things with your hands, such as sketching or doodling, working a crossword puzzle, or making a shopping list. Breathe and relax, and be thankful you are not smoking.

It is crucial for people who stop smoking to become highly skilled at handling stress. Most people who start smoking again do so when they are under increased stress. Relaxation tapes, classes, and counseling can help. Stress-reduction plans and exercises—both mental and physical—are also helpful. Use your own support system at these times. These plans for exercise and stress management are best initiated before smoking cessation, so the necessary tools will already be in place. Also, regular exercise and relaxation may reinforce the need to cut down or quit. In fact, regular exercise offers many of the same feelings smokers get from nicotine such as an "up" feeling, confidence, and a greater ability to relax and concentrate.

It is important to maintain a positive attitude and use affirmations such as "I am not a smoker" or "Stopping smoking is a great benefit to my health." Or try this, "I am not a cigarette or an ashtray. I am not supporting the greedy cigarette industry; they don't pay my health insurance." Write them down and post them in specific areas as reminders. Many ex-smokers use negative imagery to stay away from cigarettes. They think of lung damage, heart disease, wrinkled skin, or limited activity whenever they feel the urge to smoke. If we visualize these negative images when we take a deep breath and hold it, the negative feedback we feel while oxygen levels are decreasing and carbon dioxide levels are rising will help us stay off cigarettes. We should remind ourselves that we are grappling with a substance more addicting than heroin, scientifically designed to keep us involved as paying customers—then banish it! Even more important is visualizing the positive benefits, such as the new ability to taste and smell, better digestion, improved respiratory and circulatory functions, and the chance for a longer and healthier life. Increasing the love we have for ourselves as nonsmokers and continuing to see ourselves as nonsmokers are key. Every day we are not smoking, we are making progress toward improved health and better kissing!

STOP SMOKING BREW

Lemon grass	*3 parts*	*Red clover leaf*	*2 parts*	*Mullein leaf*	*2 parts*
Dandelion root	*3 parts*	*Alfalfa*	*2 parts*	*Valerian root*	*1 part*
Raspberry leaf	*2 parts*	*Peppermint*	*2 parts*	*Catnip*	*1 part*

Simmer dandelion and valerian in water for 10 minutes, then pour into a pot containing other herbs and steep for 15 minutes. Use about 1 teaspoon of root and 1 tablespoon of leaves and flowers per cup of water. Drink 1 cup several times daily or as needed for cravings.

Smoking the herbs themselves has been used to replace cigarettes temporarily or to treat bronchopulmonary problems. Mullein leaf is probably the most commonly used. Coltsfoot, yerba santa, sarsaparilla, and rosemary have also been smoked. Lobelia leaf, called "Indian tobacco," has been employed as a cigarette substitute as it acts and tastes a bit like tobacco. In China, other herbs are smoked to treat asthma and other respiratory problems. Datura leaf is sometimes used, but can be slightly toxic. Ginseng leaf and other herbal cigarettes have been available. Smoking mugwort or catnip may help in relaxation; damiana is thought to have aphrodisiac properties; peppermint added to other blends gives a cool, menthol taste and licorice adds a sweet flavor. Chewing licorice sticks replaces the oral habit and settles the system. Chewing calamus root is a nicotine version of Antabuse. Garlic (taken orally, not smoked) is also helpful during the tobacco detox period.

A program that combines other supportive therapies, including acupuncture, counseling, hypnosis and massage, with diet and supplements works wonderfully, but can be time consuming and costly. Consider adding one of these forms of support to your plan. There are a number of good smoking cessation programs available in most cities and often the cost commitment and group support add extra incentive. Avoid rapid smoking plans that make you sicker to get well, as the excessive nicotine you will ingest can be toxic. A desire to stop and the willpower to continue pursuing a non-smoking lifestyle is at the heart of all successful programs.

The nutrient levels in the following table can be spread out in several portions throughout the day. Vitamin C can be used even more frequently. The dosages range from smoker's support (low) to complete nicotine withdrawal (high), with the three to six weeks of initial detoxification requiring a mid-range amount.

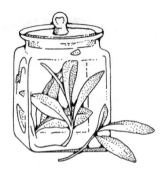

NICOTINE NUTRIENT PROGRAM

Water	2–3 qt	Copper	2–4 mg
Fat (low)	30–50 g	Iodine	150–250 mcg
Fiber	15–45 g	Iron*	women 20–30 mg
Vitamin A	5,000–10,000 IU		men 10–15 mg
Mixed carotenoids	20,000–40,000 IU	Magnesium	500–1,000 mg
Vitamin D	200–400 IU	Manganese	5–10 mg
Vitamin E	400–800 IU	Molybdenum	300–600 mcg
Vitamin K	100–300 mcg	Potassium	200–500 mg
Thiamine (B$_1$)	100–200 mg	Selenium	200–400 mcg
Riboflavin (B$_2$)	50–100 mg	Silicon	50–150 mg
Niacinamide (B$_3$)	50–100 mg	Vanadium	150–300 mcg
Niacin (B$_3$)	100–1,000 mg	Zinc	30–75 mg
Pantothenic acid (B$_5$)	250–1,000 mg	Coenzyme Q10	50–100 mg
Pyridoxine (B$_6$)	50–150 mg	L-amino acids	1,000–2,000 mg
Pyridoxal-5-phosphate	25–75 mg	L-cysteine (or NAC)	500–1,500 mg, or
Cobalamin (B$_{12}$)	200–1,000 mcg	Glutathione	250–500 mg
Folic acid	800–2,000 mcg	Glycine	250–500 mg
Biotin	200–500 mcg	Essential fatty acids	4–6 capsules
Choline	500–1,000 mg	or Flaxseed oil	2–3 teaspoons
PABA	500–1,500 mg		
Vitamin C	3–12 g	**For Withdrawal and Detox:**	
Bioflavonoids	250–750 mg	Garlic	3–6 capsules
Quercetin	400 mg	Valerian root	4–6 capsules
Calcium	850–1,250 mg	Lobelia leaf	1–2 capsules
Chromium	200–500 mcg	Carrot sticks	10–20

*levels depend on body needs and blood loss.

NICOTINE DETOX SUMMARY

1. Eat an alkaline diet of fruits, vegetables, and whole grains. Follow the Detox Diet, or try a vegetarian or raw foods diet during detox. Reduce acid foods and potential carcinogens, such as fats, food additives, and alcohol.

2. Drink 2 to 3 quarts of pure water a day.

3. Keep fiber intake high to support detoxification and colon function.

4. Maintain vitamin levels through supplementation (see previous page). If cravings are strong, take 1 gram of vitamin C every 1 to 2 hours.

5. Also, take sodium or potassium bicarbonate tablets to alkalinize your body—1 for each occasion of craving, but not more than 6 daily.

6. Use herbal supplements, including herbal stop-smoking brews.

7. Exercise, especially in the fresh air, to oxygenate your body.

8. If you are having real difficulty stopping, consider the use of nicotine patches or gum to help your transition.

9. Use acupuncture or hypnosis to motivate you to stop and/or to support you in withdrawal and detox.

10. Ease detox with relaxing therapies—hot baths or showers, saunas or hot tubs, swimming, and massage.

11. Practice relaxation and deep breathing. Get to know nature.

12. Build a method of support into your plan, including friends, family, and counseling. Stay busy and know that you are taking care of yourself, especially for the future.

13. Find oral substitutes for smoking. Change daily patterns to avoid smoking stimuli.

14. Do a journal/tape review of how and when you were first influenced to smoke. Evaluate the focus of your new and previous relationship to smoking.

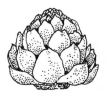

SCOPE OF THE NICOTINE PROBLEM

Tobacco use is the leading preventable cause of disease and premature death in the United States—430,000 deaths annually.

The U.S. government estimates approximately 400,000 annual premature deaths due to cigarette smoking (1998).

Over 70 percent of tobacco associated deaths will occur in the developing world.

Current Tobacco Use

In 1999, 67 million Americans smoked cigarettes.

This represents 30 percent among the U.S. population age 12 and older.

Males are more likely than females to report the use of any tobacco product.

Mortality Rates

The past 25 years has been marked by a steady decline in cigarette consumption.

Tobacco use contributes to 1 in every 5 deaths.

A 35-year-old male who smokes 2 packs a day has a life expectancy that is 8.1 years shorter than his nonsmoking counterpart.

Tobacco Use Without Smoking—Dipping, Chewing, and Snuffing

In 1999, 7.6 million Americans used smokeless tobacco.

The prevalence of smokeless tobacco use is increasing.

Increased risk of oral cancer.

Secondhand and Sidestream Smoke Definitions

Mainstream smoke—smoke drawn through the mouthpiece of the cigarette.

Passive smoking—nonsmokers' inhalation of tobacco smoke.

Environmental tobacco smoke—sidestream smoke and exhaled mainstream smoke that is inhaled by the passive smoker.

Current smokers are more likely to be heavy drinkers and illicit drug users.

Highest rate of smokers is among 18 to 25 year olds.

College graduates are the least likely to smoke.

Methods for Quitting

"Cold turkey"

Behavioral modification

Smoking cessation aids:

Nicotine gum	Nicotine inhalers
Nicotine patches	Buproprion (Wellbutrin)
Nicotine nasal spray	

Major Conclusions of the Surgeon General's Report about Women

- Despite all that is known of the devastating health consequences of smoking, 22 percent of women smoked cigarettes in 1998. Cigarette smoking became prevalent among men first, and smoking in the United States has always been lower among women than among men. However, the once-wide gender gap in smoking narrowed until the mid-1980s and has since remained fairly constant. Smoking today is nearly three times higher among women who have only nine to eleven years of education (32.9 percent) than among women with sixteen or more years of education (11.2 percent).

- In 2000, 29.7 percent of high school senior girls reported having smoked within the past thirty days. Smoking among white girls declined from the mid-1970s to the early 1980s, followed by a decade of little change. Smoking then increased markedly in the early 1990s and declined somewhat in the late 1990s. The increase dampened much of the earlier progress. Among black girls, smoking declined substantially from the mid-1970s to the early 1990s, followed by some increases until the mid-1990s. Data on long-term trends in smoking among high school seniors of other racial or ethnic groups are not available.

- Since 1980, approximately 3 million U.S. women have died prematurely from smoking-related neoplastic, cardiovascular, and respiratory diseases. Each year during the 1990s, U.S. women lost an estimated 2.1 million years of life due to these smoking-attributable premature deaths. In Addition, women who smoke experience gender-specific health consequences, including increased risk of various adverse reproductive outcomes.

- Lung cancer is now the leading cause of cancer death among U.S. women; it surpassed breast cancer in 1987. About 90 percent of all lung cancer deaths among women who continue to smoke are attributable to smoking.

- Exposure to environmental tobacco smoke is a cause of lung cancer and coronary heart disease among women who are lifetime nonsmokers. Infants born to women exposed to environmental tobacco smoke during pregnancy have a small decrease in birth weight and a slightly increased risk of intrauterine growth retardation compared with infants of non-exposed women.

- Women who stop smoking greatly reduce their risk of dying prematurely, and quitting smoking is beneficial at all ages. Women may have more difficulty quitting smoking than men, yet a national survey data show that women are quitting at rates similar to or even higher than those for men. Prevention and cessation interventions are generally of similar effectiveness for women and men, and, to date, few gender differences in factors related to smoking initiation and successful quitting have been identified.

- Smoking during pregnancy remains a major public health problem despite increased knowledge of the adverse health effects of smoking during pregnancy. Although smoking during pregnancy has declined steadily in recent years, substantial numbers of pregnant women continue to smoke, and only about one-third of women who stop smoking during pregnancy are still abstinent 1 year after the delivery.

- Tobacco industry marketing is a factor influencing susceptibility to and initiation of smoking among girls in the United States and overseas. Myriad examples of tobacco ads and promotions targeted to women indicate that such marketing is dominated by themes of social desirability and independence. These themes are conveyed through ads featuring slim, attractive, and athletic models, images very much at odds with the serious health consequences experienced by so many women who smoke.

CHAPTER NINE

Alcohol Detoxification

♦

Even though alcohol is enjoyed worldwide and has been used for thousands of years, its regular overconsumption poses a serious health hazard. As with caffeine, occasional or moderate use is often pleasurable and is no cause for concern except for people with allergic reactions to alcohol or diseases of the liver, gastrointestinal tract, kidneys, brain, or nervous system. Habitual alcohol over-consumption, however, can lead to addiction, emotional problems, and a number of specific degenerative processes including obesity, gastritis and ulcers, hepatitis, cirrhosis, pancreatitis, hypoglycemia and diabetes, gout, nerve and brain dysfunction, cancer, nutritional deficiencies, immune suppression, accidental injury, and death. Most people can handle periodic use, but for many others, it is a significant problem.

Alcohol does have some positive physiological effects. It stimulates the appetite and relieves stress, although not as much as exercise. It acts as a vasodilator, improving blood flow. Alcohol may also affect a slight increase in HDL "good" cholesterol levels, however it also raises total blood fats. Small to moderate amounts (one to two drinks daily) may also lessen the progression of atherosclerosis and heart disease. Some studies have shown a lower number of heart attacks in moderate drinkers over non-drinkers of the same age, possibly due to increased HDL cholesterol levels and reduced atherosclerosis. Higher amounts of alcohol, however, increase blood pressure and heart disease risk. More research is needed to understand the real link between alcohol (and the chemicals used) and heart disease before prescribing it as a preventative measure. Certainly regular physical activity and nurturing personal relationships are better health supporters and stress reducers than alcohol.

There are over 100 million regular drinkers in the United States alone and about 11 million who report heavy alcohol use. More than half of our population is composed of social drinkers (138 million). Social drinking and problem drinking mean different things to different people. If you feel that alcohol is a problem for you, consider the following: "For every alcoholic, there are four problem drinkers," says Mark Sobell, a professor at the center for psychological studies at Nova Southeastern University. He estimates there are 12 million problem drinkers in the United States. Alcoholism, now considered a disease by the American Medical Association, occurs when one becomes physically dependent upon alcohol.

Problem or excessive drinkers average twelve or more drinks per week or binge at least five times a year. Bingeing is defined as consuming five or more drinks at a time. Alcohol is a particularly big concern for our youth. More and more children are trying alcohol, and in 1992, an estimated 5 percent of children ages twelve to seventeen consumed alcohol more than fifty days during that year.

Sobell and his wife, Linda, also an NSU psychology professor, conducted a yearlong study of 825 problem drinkers who wanted to cut back. They discovered participants who received generic educational pamphlets cut down their weekly intake on average by 15 percent to 33 percent.

The costs of alcohol abuse to human lives and the economy are enormous. According to the latest reports gathered by the National Institute on Alcohol Abuse and Alcoholism, each year alcohol abuse in the United States is responsible for $134 billion in lost productivity, including $87 billion in losses from alcohol-related illness, $36 billion in premature death, and $10 billion in crime.

Yearly health-care expenses for treating alcohol-related illnesses include more than $7 billion spent in direct treatment and $19 billion spent on the treatment of medical consequences. Alcohol-related vehicle crashes cost the country more than $15 billion a year, while the criminal justice system spends more than $6 billion on alcohol-related crime. Those statistics might be sharply reduced if mass mailings of educational materials would be sent to problem drinkers, says Sobell.

The Sobells' study was published in the June 1992 issue of *Alcoholism: Clinical and Experimental Research*, the official journal of the Research Society on Alcoholism and the International Society for Biomedical Research on Alcoholism.

EMPTY CALORIES MEAN INSUFFICIENT NUTRITION

Alcohol is a source of empty calories; it contains seven of them per gram, almost double the calories found in regular carbohydrates and protein (four calories per gram each). The average social drinker consumes 5 to 10 percent of his or her calories from alcohol, while heavy drinkers may consume more than 50 percent in place of real nutrition.

Since alcohol is replacing regular nutrition, the body receives decreased amounts of essential vitamins, minerals, and other nutrients, causing deficiencies over time. In addition, the alcohol molecule is so small and easy to absorb that it gets assimilated before other foods, directly entering the bloodstream for a quick effect. Beer, wine, and mixed drinks cause rapid fluctuations of the blood sugar with accompanying mood swings.

The liver is the only organ that metabolizes alcohol, either converting it into energy or storing it as fat when there is excess consumption. When stored as fat, alcohol acts as a liver irritant and can eventually lead to cirrhosis or scarring of the liver tissue. About 5 percent of ingested alcohol is eliminated through sweat, urine, and breath.

Many people think of alcohol as a stimulant because it reduces inhibitions and, in small amounts, seems to ease and enhance social interactions. It is actually a sedative that depresses the central nervous system. The effects are pleasantly tranquilizing at first. However, with continued consumption the calming effect deteriorates into mental and physical numbness, hampering our reflexes, coordination, and judgment. This is why there are so many alcohol-related accidents both while walking and driving.

Despite all these problems, alcohol is rooted in our culture. For centuries alcohol was used as an anesthetic to treat physical pain. Nowadays it is used to anesthetize emotional pain. Alcohol abuse and alcoholism are clearly diseases that involve genetics, social/cultural values, and environmental influences and that have emotional consequences. It is possible that it may involve an enzyme deficiency or be linked to a deficiency or improper function of chromium (a trace mineral related to blood sugar metabolism). Whatever its cause, problems related to alcohol abuse definitely seem to run in families.

Alcohol drinks can also be allergenic as they contain grains, grapes, sugar, and yeast, producing both intestinal and cerebral symptoms. Corn, wheat, rye, and barley can also cause allergic reactions. Alcoholism may even be an advanced food addiction in which the allergens themselves stimulate addiction; in such cases, withdrawal from the offending food produces uncomfortable psychological and physical symptoms. Alcohol products are also problematic for people with a yeast overgrowth in the body (especially intestines), as it feeds the yeast and stimulates its growth. Furthermore, many people react to various chemicals, such as sulfites, which are used in manufacturing alcohol.

It has been suggested that alcohol is a viable source of nourishment. Wine does contain vitamin C from grape or rice juice, yet it also contains 9 to 12 percent alcohol (empty calories). In sherry and port wine, alcohol content may be as high as 12 to 18 percent. Beer and ale contain B vitamins and minerals from the cereal grains and yeast, with a range from 3 to 6 percent alcohol. Alcohol distillates or "spirits" such as gin, vodka, rum, and whiskey are also made from grain products. These range from 35 to 50 percent alcohol—that is, 70 to 100 proof. In reality, none of these beverages are very nourishing when calorie levels are compared with nutrient levels.

RISKS OF ALCOHOL

The risk levels of alcohol are directly related to the amount consumed and the time period over which it is used, although individual reactions may vary. High-risk use involves more than five drinks daily; moderate-risk use, three to five drinks daily; and low-risk, one or two. Social drinking of a few drinks a week offers minimal risk.

Those with diabetes, hypertension, or heart disease, and pregnant or nursing mothers, or those planning pregnancy should not drink alcohol at all. People with

CALORIE CONTENT OF ALCOHOLIC BEVERAGES

Amount that Provides 0.5 oz of Alcohol	Type of Beverage	Calories
1 oz	100 or 110 proof liquor	80
1½ oz	80 proof liquor	90–110
5 oz	8–10 percent wine (French, German)	100
4 oz	12–14 percent wine (most American)	95
3 oz	17–20 percent wine (sherry, port)	80
2½ oz	18 percent dessert wine	120
8 oz	6–7 percent dark beer (stout, porter)	150
12 oz	4.5 percent regular beer	140
12 oz	light beer	90
6 oz	mixed drinks (juices, sodas, sweeteners)	100–250

blood sugar problems, liver disorders (especially hepatitis), ulcers and gastritis, viral diseases, yeast problems, mental confusion, fatigue, or hypersensitive reactions to alcoholic beverages should also avoid it.

Symptoms from drinking include dizziness, delayed reflexes, slowed mental functions, memory loss, poor judgment, emotional outburst, aggressive behavior, lack of coordination, and loss of consciousness. Symptoms of hangover include mouth dryness, thirst, headache, throbbing temples, nausea, vomiting, stomach upset, fatigue, and dizziness. Alcohol dehydrates the cells, removes fluid from the blood, swells the cranial arteries, and irritates the gastrointestinal tract. Hangovers are more common with stronger, distilled alcohol drinks but can still occur with red and white wines, champagne, and beer.

Symptoms of withdrawal include alcohol craving, nausea, vomiting, gastrointestinal upset, abdominal cramps, dehydration, anorexia, fatigue, headache, anxiety, irritability, dizziness, fevers, chills, depression, insomnia, tremors, weakness, hallucinations, and seizures.

Drinking can put us at risk to inadvertently harm ourselves or others. Alcohol is involved in the more than 25,000 auto accident deaths yearly. About 20 percent of home accidental deaths are attributed to alcohol plus alcohol-related domestic violence.

Ninety-five percent of alcohol consumed must be metabolized in the liver, taking precedence over other functions. Fat metabolism slows and fat builds up in the liver. Since alcohol converts to fat, obesity (especially abdominal obesity, the most dangerous area) also often occurs with high alcohol use. Chronic use can swell, scar, and shrink the liver, until only a small percentage is functional. Complications also include ascites (fluid buildup in the abdomen), hemorrhoids, varicose veins, and bleeding disorders. More serious liver disease such as hepatitis and cirrhosis, when the liver becomes inflamed or enlarged, are also the result of chronic alcohol use. Usually more than half the liver must be destroyed before its work is significantly impaired (but it can regenerate if drinking is stopped).

Gastrointestinal disorders include gastritis, abdominal pain, eating difficulties, gastric ulcers, duodenal ulcers, deficiency of hydrochloric acid and digestive enzymes, "leaky gut" syndrome, esophagitis (irritation of the esophagus), varicose veins, pancreatitis, gallstones, and gall bladder disease.

Alcohol can cross the blood-brain barrier, destroying brain cells and causing brain damage and behavioral and psychological problems; nervous system disorders, including polyneuritis (nerve inflammations), premature senility, and encephalopathy (chronic degenerative brain syndrome) can also result from chronic alcohol use.

Although modest alcohol intake may, in fact, raise HDL cholesterol and protect against atherosclerosis, the effect of alcohol abuse on the heart and blood vessels is damaging and leads to cardiovascular diseases and dysfunctions. These include a decrease in heart function, heart muscle action, and electrical conductivity, congestive heart failure, cardiac arrythmias, and an enlarged heart.

Carbohydrate metabolism is affected by alcohol and can lead to hypoglycemia and diabetes. Alcohol is a simple sugar that is rapidly absorbed and has a tendency to weaken glucose tolerance with chronic use. Impaired glucose metabolism can cause mood swings, depression, emotional outbursts, or anxiety. Furthermore, increased calories from alcohol can lead to weight gain and increased body fat resulting in obesity as alcohol converts to fat unless it is balanced by exercise and a good diet.

Nutritional deficiencies from alcohol use potentially include impaired absorption of nutrients, particularly B vitamins and minerals; liver impairment from reduced absorption of the fat-soluble vitamins A, D, E, and K; loss of nutrients like potassium and magnesium from alcohol's diuretic effect; reduced liver stores of alcohol-metabolizing vitamins B_1 and B_3; anemia due to deficiency of folic acid, vitamin B_{12}, and iron; increased risk of osteoporosis from low vitamin D and poor calcium absorption; lack of appetite, causing deficiencies in vitamin B_2, B_6, A, C, essential fatty acids, methionine, or really any nutrient that comes from a good and wholesome diet.

Alcohol increases levels of the liver enzyme that breaks down testosterone. In teenage boys, the reduction of testosterone may delay sexual maturity. Alcohol's depressant effect on the nervous system can reduce sexual performance or cause impotence despite reduced inhibitions and increased desire.

Alcohol has been implicated in malignancies of the mouth, esophagus, pancreas, and breasts. Cigarette smoke and alcohol combined are thought to create ethyl nitrite, which is a strong mutagen. Other health problems include a red swollen nose, dilated blood vessels, gout, yeast vaginitis, PMS, and a suppressed immune system. Because alcohol crosses the placenta and enters fetal circulation, fetal alcohol syndrome results in undersized babies often with mental deficits due to brain damage. There is no "safe" level of alcohol intake—women who are pregnant should simply not drink! Regular alcohol use and abuse can create social problems in personal relationships and career, and economic adversity in regard to lost work and medical costs.

ALCOHOLISM

The alcoholic is someone who has lost control over the drug. Research suggests that there is a genetic component to problem drinking. An intense biological craving for alcohol or the products from which it is made might be at the root, as might problems with blood sugar metabolism or allergy-addictions. The ability to easily stop drinking for a week or two at a time is a good sign. Remember, many people with a drinking problem deny that there is one. Warning signs of alcoholism include drinking alone, drinking in place of meals, drinking before social or business functions, drinking in the morning or late at night, missing work because of drinking, and periods of amnesia or blackouts. People who have these concerns should definitely seek help.

Once we've admitted that we need outside resources to deal with alcohol, it is important to get the support of our spouse or a friend. Clear the alcohol from all areas of life (home, work, car, and so on), and then see a physician or therapist. A medical check-up with laboratory testing may be in order. Some cases require tranquilizers during the first few days of withdrawal. With a multilevel approach combining community and professional support, the chances of recovery from alcohol are better than 50 percent.

Psychological counseling, family therapy, Alcoholics Anonymous (AA), or religious/spiritual practices may also improve our motivation, self-image, and ability to create a new life. AA meetings continue the positive support for many recovering alcoholics. Avoiding negative influences such as old drinking buddies and exposure to alcohol is also helpful. Regular exercise is valuable, especially at the usual drinking time. In addition, weight training is an excellent way to work off stress and anger. Learning and practicing relaxation exercises can also be useful. Massage therapy promotes relaxation and self-love. Acupuncture is usually beneficial during withdrawal and detox, as it seems to reduce the stress from cravings and other symptoms that may reappear periodically after the initial detox process.

The amount of time it takes to detoxify from alcohol depends on the level of abuse, and it may take months or even years to completely clear its effects. Mild withdrawal symptoms include increased tension, headaches, and irritability for a few days. Medical care in a hospital setting is not uncommon for acute alcohol withdrawal, although this is usually necessary only for those who consume more than six to eight drinks daily.

ALCOHOL
by Bethany Argisle

Everyone seemed to have had some
  It seemed part of the lifestyle
  It was advertised, offered and refilled
  It influenced my first sensual explorations
  Is it that we need something to uninhibit us out of ourselves, which
is all we know ever no matter what?

That is why I drank, to get away with being myself. And, as a teen I
got away with my secret consumptions and my underage purchasing of
Southern Comfort on the rocks, which leaked from the soles of my
argyle socks. Things began disappearing, especially my self-respect and
consciousness. To this day, I enjoy a few well-planned ceremonial times
to let go and enjoy a moment—but not all of the time like previously.
It became a lifestyle that I could not escape from until I had a horrid
car accident. Did that stop me? Only for a while, I still didn't get the
connection.

Of course, I was working in an industry that needed to do something
to relieve the constant pressure that produced one of the top daily major
metropolitan newspapers. There were always cocktail parties, drinks
after work—I never thought much about harm being done to me, my
brain, my abilities to reflex and respond. More drinks? Sure! Two mar-
tinis, why not four?

That full glass; was the atmosphere of the career, and accomplishing
so much and having another round for the town at the same time. They
had drinks everywhere—it's a miracle I made it—and I have spent years
of tears, time, and money cleansing my liver, my giver of life.

Yet when ritual becomes habit, alcohol eventually eats up your ability
to judge distance and time, self and one another.

In 1980 when Elson and I traveled to do a health convention in
Santa Fe, New Mexico, we took some time after the event and drove to
the ancient Taos Pueblo area. We found ourselves in the ancient square,
going into buildings that are made of the Earth, had no electricity,
opened with the sun in the marketplace and closed with the sun and
moon exchanging places. Here is where I met saints and alcoholics.
The alcohol situation permeated nations of peoples (especially Native
Americans) who still suffer. It seems alcohol suffering occurs with long-

term use, especially if you are one who cannot tolerate this type of toxin. Detoxification is part of the plan to regain your health.

Alcohol at the extreme is the outcome of a very bad body dream. However, a bit of wine with dinner can be a winner. I say this because I live in and occasionally enjoy the wine country.

The use of alcohol has to do with the use of your faculties to choose what is wise, what is real, what leads to what, and how you are going to fuel your health or your demise.

Never drink alcohol when you are caring for children; I have seen this lead to accusations of every kind and some of them are true. You must never drink and drive or drive with anyone who is that way. Keep track of where you are placing your body at all times.

NO is ON backwards. And this pertains to drugs of all kinds, and junk foods.

I still drink some alcoholic beverages, and enjoy them when I do. Water, however, is my main drink. Make sure you have your daily share. Instead of reaching for a glass, I reach for my drum and the beat. Through healthier choices, I discovered that my life is a prayer devoted to who I am. Let life be allowed to unfold—not inside of a glass, inside of your heartbeat.

If willpower is poor, drugs such as Antabuse (disulfiram), which produce terrible nausea and vomiting when alcohol is used, can be a powerful deterrent. Antabuse is usually fairly well tolerated for a short time, but it can have side effects on the cardiovascular system and psyche. Lithium therapy has recently been shown to reduce the urge to drink. For recovering alcoholics, I believe that it is imperative to avoid all alcohol for life, because the addictive potential never disappears. Nonalcoholic beverages may be fine, but even some de-alcoholized drinks contain small amounts of the drug.

ALCOHOL DETOXIFICATION

Diet and megavitamin therapy are helpful during withdrawal, detoxification, and recovery. Certainly, people who use alcohol excessively need more supplements than others, and during detox they may require even more. During the actual withdrawal period, diet should focus on fluids and alkaline foods. The appetite is usually not very strong at this time; liquids are easy to consume and will also help clear alcohol from the body. Water, diluted fruit and vegetable juices, warm broths, soups, and teas using herbs such as chamomile, skullcap (a nervine), or valerian root are good choices. Other helpful herbs include white willow bark for reducing pain and inflammation, ginseng, cayenne, and peppermint. Small amounts of light proteins, such as non-fatty poultry, fish, or even chicken soup will provide more nourishment. Amino acid powder is also supportive. L-glutamine, an amino acid, has been shown to reduce cravings for alcohol and sugar, and is used in many detox clinics.

I have seen intravenous supplements work quite well during withdrawal. Extra vitamin C, B complex, and minerals such as calcium, magnesium, and potassium, can be used intravenously, especially if supplements taken by mouth are not well tolerated. Vitamin C powder buffered with these minerals and mixed into water or juice is helpful during withdrawal and later during the detox period.

Alcohol detoxification continues for several weeks after withdrawal. During this recovery time, the body will eliminate alcohol, its by-products, and other toxins, and begin breaking down some of the stored fat. Balanced nourishment with a low-fat, moderate-protein, complex-carbohydrate diet is recommended. Since alcoholics often have blood sugar problems, basic hypoglycemic principles should also be followed. These include avoiding sugars and refined foods such as soft drinks or candy, and eating every few hours. The basic diet consists of small meals and snacks of protein or complex carbohydrates including whole grains, pasta, potatoes, squashes, legumes, and other vegetables. Proteins such as soy products, sprouted beans, some nuts or seeds, eggs, fish, or poultry can also be added, and small amounts of fruits and fruit juices may be tolerated. Since the primary aim is to maintain an alkaline diet, we should initially focus on vegetables and fruit. Of course, the Detox Diet can be used during the first two weeks of alcohol detoxification.

Water or herbal teas should be consumed throughout the day. Foods containing potentially damaging fats such as fast foods, lunch meats, chips, burgers, hot dogs, and ice cream should also be avoided, as they are all congesting and more acid-forming. Caffeine consumption and cigarette smoking are best minimized. Many people recovering from alcohol addiction consume large amounts of coffee and smoke intensely—an event seen clearly at some AA meetings. I do not recommend this at all. Fortunately, there has been an increase in the number of nonsmoking AA meetings and in general, many people are aware of improving all health habits during recovery.

During detoxification from alcohol, as with the other substances, supplemental nutrients are helpful. Herbal formulas, such as valerian root capsules, or prescription medicines can be used for sleep. Calcium and magnesium supplements taken at night may also aid sleep. L-glutamine, an amino acid that generates glutamic acid, can be used for energy. Glutamine is found naturally in liver, meats, dairy foods, and cabbage, and helps diminish the craving for alcohol and sugar. A supplement amount of 500 to 1,000 mg three times daily between or before meals is suggested, either in capsule or powdered form. Chromium may also help with sugar and alcohol cravings, at 200 mcg twice daily. Melatonin can also be used and has had some good effects during detox for aiding sleep. One 3-mg tablet (the sublingual variety is best) can be taken at bedtime.

A multiple vitamin with additional antioxidant nutrients is a good idea during detox from alcohol. Minerals such as zinc, iron, calcium, and magnesium should be taken to replace those lost during alcohol abuse. Higher levels of niacin, even up to 2 grams, along with 5 to 10 grams of vitamin C daily have been used with some success in alcohol withdrawal and detox. For basic support, vitamin C intake would be 500 to 1,000 mg taken four to six times daily.

Fiber helps bind toxins in the bowel and improve elimination. Choline and inositol, in doses of about 500 mg each three times daily, will improve fat digestion and utilization. Lemon water combined with a couple of teaspoons of olive oil and a quarter teaspoon or capsule of cayenne pepper will help detoxify the liver. You can decrease the oil absorption by taking fiber along with it, but olive oil alone is also thought to be nourishing to the liver and helpful in clearing chemical toxins. Cold-pressed olive oil is commonly used in many natural liver therapies. Milk thistle herb (Silybum marianum or Silymarin) offers protection and healing to the liver in detoxification; taking between 60 and 100 mg twice daily is suggested. Taking one or two capsules of goldenseal root powder twice daily is also helpful for toning and cleaning the liver. Parsley tea improves kidney elimination and cleanses the blood. The amino acid L-cysteine is another helpful detoxicant for the liver, blood, and colon.

Other nutrients and herbs can also be helpful. These include pancreatic digestive enzymes, taken after meals, and Brewer's yeast if tolerated, which supplies many B vitamins and minerals. The essential fatty acids help decrease the inflammatory prostaglandins. Gamma-linolenic acid from evening primrose or borage seed oil assists in the reduction of alcohol toxicity. White willow bark tablets can be used for pain, and valerian root, a natural and milder form of Valium, can be taken to decrease anxiety. Chamomile will help calm the digestive tract, as will licorice root.

NUTRITIONAL SUPPORT FOR DRINKERS

The basic support plan for active drinkers resembles that which is used during complete alcohol detox. A generally balanced and nutritious diet will help minimize some of the potential problems from alcohol, although even the best diet and supplement program will not fully protect us from ethanol's toxic effects. When our liver is metabolizing alcohol, it is helpful to avoid fried foods, rancid or hydrogenated fats, and other drugs, all of which are hard on the liver. Alpha-lipoic (thioctic) acid may help protect the liver against some of the toxicity, as can milk thistle herb.

Alcohol users need more nutrients than most people to protect them from malnutrition. Obviously, basic multivitamins and antioxidant formulas are important. Part, or possibly most of, the toxic effects of alcohol may be caused by the production of free radicals. Higher-than-DRI (Daily Recommended Index) levels of vitamins A, C, and E, mixed carotenes, and the minerals selenium, zinc, manganese, and magnesium are suggested (for all dosages, see supplement table, page xxx). Commonly deficient nutrients also need extra support. Thiamine, riboflavin, and niacin help circulation and blood cleansing and can reduce the effects of hangovers. I recommend folic acid in an amount more than twice the DRI can be taken; leafy greens and whole grains, both rich in this vitamin, should be added to the diet.

Water and other nonalcoholic liquids are needed to counteract the dehydrating effects of alcohol. Calcium is supportive, as is extra zinc, as its absorption is diminished and elimination is increased with alcohol use. This supplemental intake should be balanced out with copper. The essential fatty acids and gamma-linolenic acid from evening primrose oil or borage seed oil support normal fat metabolism and protect against inflammation caused by free radicals and prostaglandins (PGEs). Alcohol decreases the levels of the anti-inflammatory PGE_1, and these oils will begin to raise their levels again. Glutathione helps prevent fat buildup in the liver through its enzymatic activities, so the tripeptide glutathione (or L-cysteine, which forms glutathione in the body) may be supplemented along with basic L-amino acids. Additional L-glutamine will enhance brain cell function.

Social Drinking

I recommend that social drinkers use a lighter version of this program, as they still need protection against alcohol's toxicity. A good diet is, of course, essential, plus vitamins B_1, B_2, and B_3, folic acid, and B_{12}. These, along with zinc (15 to 30 mg), magnesium (300 to 500 mg), and vitamin C (1,000 mg) should be taken with some food before drinking. In general, drinking should be limited to two drinks per day.

A number of things can help prevent drunkenness and hangover. Our alcohol blood level is affected by how much and how fast we drink and absorb. Drink slowly. If we drink fast on an empty stomach, absorption is immediate. Ideally, it is best to have some food in the stomach or to limit consumption to one drink before eating. Food also prevents us from getting sick. We recommend low-salt complex carbohydrates such as whole-grain bread, crackers, or vegetable sticks, because carbohydrates delay alcohol absorption. Fat-protein snacks such as milk or cheese will also decrease alcohol absorption, thus reducing drunkenness and hangovers. Some people even drink a little olive oil before parties to coat their stomachs before drinking. A few capsules of evening primrose oil will have a similar effect. Women seem to be more readily affected by alcohol than men, even when body weight is equal.

Once alcohol is ingested, it just takes time to clear it from the blood. With heavy drinking, extra coffee and exercise do not really help; however, with mild intoxication they can increase alertness. Definitely avoid other psychoactive drugs when drinking alcohol, including tranquilizers, narcotics, sedatives, antihistamines, and marijuana, all of which may increase alcohol's effect.

Alcohol blood levels have been studied in order to understand their varying effect. Tests are used to clarify degrees of safety while under the influence, versus more potentially dangerous drunkenness. Usually one or two drinks will leave people in the safe range, but more can create problems. Hangovers are caused both by the dehydrating effect of alcohol and by the toxic effects of the chemical congeners or sulfur compounds created during fermentation or added to the beverages. Allergies to some of the ingredients such as corn, wheat, barley, or yeast may intensify hangovers and withdrawal.

Alcohol Blood Level	Status Typical Experience
0.05 percent	"Cruising," feeling good, some positive effects
0.05–0.1	Beginning loss of balance, speech, or emotions
0.08	Legally drunk
0.2	Passed out
0.3	Comatose, unresponsive

The best hangover remedy is to prevent them altogether by not overdrinking and taking supportive fluids and nutrients. Cream, coffee, oysters, chili peppers, and aspirin are common and occasionally helpful hangover remedies. Time is the only real remedy, however, along with rest and fluids. If alcohol intake has been excessive, drink two or three glasses of water before going to bed, along with some vitamin C and a B complex vitamin to clear alcohol from the blood. Repeat upon awakening. Emergen-C can also be used—it is a vitamin C powder with added vitamins and minerals, and is available at natural food stores. Evening primrose oil and flaxseed oil also help. A morning-after plan suggested by Dr. Stuart Berger includes 100 mg of thiamine, 100 mg of riboflavin, 50 mg of B_6, 250 mcg of B_{12}, 1,000 mg of vitamin C, and 50 mg of zinc.

Overall, we need to monitor our drinking and not let alcohol use turn into abuse and addiction. We also need to pay special attention to children and teenagers and offer them education regarding alcohol and drugs and provide them with good role models in ourselves. Let us all live as examples of how we would like the world to be.

ALCOHOL NUTRIENT PROGRAMS			
	Support	Withdrawal	Detox/Recovery
Water	2½–3 qt	3–4 qt	3 qt
Protein	60–80 g	50–70 g	75–100 g
Fats and Oils	30–50 g	30–50 g	50–65 g
Fiber	15–20 g	10–15 g	30–40 g
Vitamin A	10,000 IU	5,000 IU	10,000 IU
Beta or mixed carotenes	25,000 IU	20,000 IU	20,000 IU
Vitamin D	200 IU	400 IU	400 IU
Vitamin E	400-800 IU	400 IU	800 IU
Vitamin K	300 mcg	300 mcg	500 mcg
Thiamine (B_1)	100 mg	50–100 mg	150 mg
Riboflavin (B_2)	100 mg	50–100 mg	150 mg
Niacinamide (B_3)	50 mg	50 mg	50 mg
Niacin (B_3)	50–150 mg	100–1,000 mg	200–2,000 mg
Pantothenic acid (B_5)	250 mg	1,000 mg	500 mg
Pyridoxine (B_6)	100 mg	200 mg	100 mg
Pyridoxal-5-phosphate	50 mg	100 mg	50 mg

	Support	Withdrawal	Detox/Recovery
COBALAMIN (B$_{12}$)	100 MCG	200 MCG	250 MCG
Folic acid	800–1,000 mcg	2,000 mcg	800 mcg
Biotin	300 mcg	500 mcg	500 mcg
Choline	500 mg	1,000 mg	1,500 mg
Inositol	500 mg	1,000 mg	1,500 mg
Vitamin C	2–4 g	5–25 g	5–10 g
Bioflavonoids	250 mg	500 mg	500 mg
Calcium*	850–1,000 mg	1,000–1,500 mg	1,000 mg
Chromium	500 mcg	500-1,000 mcg	300 mcg
Copper*	3 mg	3 mg	3–4 mg
Iodine	150 mcg	150 mcg	150 mcg
Iron*	15–30 mg	10–18 mg	20 mg
Magnesium*	500–800 mg	800–1,000 mg	600–800 mg
Manganese	5 mg	15 mg	10 mg
Molybdenum	300 mcg	300 mcg	300 mcg
Potassium*	300–500 mg	500 mg	300 mg
Selenium	300 mcg	150 mcg	200 mcg
Silicon	100 mg	50 mg	200 mg
Vanadium	150 mcg	150 mcg	150 mcg
Zinc*	45–75 mg	50–75 mg	50–100 mg
Flaxseed oil	1 teaspoon	2 teaspoons	2 teaspoons
Gamma-linolenic acid (40-60 mg/capsule)	3 capsules	3 capsules	6 capsules
L-amino acids	1,000–1,500 mg	1,500–3,000 mg	5,000–7,500 mg
L-glutamine	500–1,000 mg	1,500–3,000 mg	1,000–2,000 mg
Lipoic acid	100 mg	100 mg	200 mg
L-cysteine or	250 mg	250 mg	250–500 mg
Glutathione	250 mg	500 mg	250 mg
Digestive enzymes	—	—	1–2 after meals
Goldenseal root	—	—	3 capsules
White willow bark (for pain)	1–2 tablets	4–6 tablets	2–4 tablets
Silymarin (milk thistle) (60–80 mg caps or tabs)	2–4 capsules	3 capsules	3–6 capsules

*Amounts may vary based on individual needs.

ALCOHOL DETOX SUMMARY

1. If you have been drinking for a long time or drink large amounts, seek multi-leveled support. This gives you the best chance for a permanent change. Also, have some professional support and guidance for this process.

2. If you consume more than 6 to 8 drinks daily, seriously consider inpatient help or a residential detox program.

3. The Juice Cleanse or the Detox Diet, often accompanied with light protein and amino acids, can be useful in the transition and detox process. Post-detox, whole foods with complex carbohydrates and adequate proteins can be nourishing.

4. Follow basic hypoglycemic guidelines—avoid sugars and sweetened foods, have some nourishment regularly (every 2 to 3 hours), and maintain adequate protein intake.

5. Drink 6 to 8 glasses or more of water daily to help clear the liver and cleanse the body of toxins.

6. Include sufficient fiber to support proper bowel elimination.

7. Use nutritional supplements to support your body during detoxification from alcohol. Medically supervised intravenous (IV) nutrition of vitamins B and C along with minerals may also be useful.

8. Be sure to include antioxidant nutrients to help with detox—namely, vitamins C and E, beta-carotene, zinc, and selenium.

9. Use specific herbs to cleanse and heal the liver and facilitate detoxification—these include milk thistle (silymarin), dandelion root, and others.

10. Consider acupuncture to treat physical cravings and withdrawal symptoms.

11. Get support that fits your own values—perhaps psychological counseling, family therapy, AA, or a religious or spiritual practice.

12. Avoid places and people that most trigger your drinking.

13. Evaluate yourself—when and how were you first introduced to drinking. When did it become a problem both emotionally and physically? Keep a journal so you can track your personal process.

CHAPTER TEN

Caffeine Detoxification

◆

Caffeine is a worldwide ubiquitous drug. Used originally in most cultures for ceremonies, it has become an overused energy stimulant in the Western world with the United States leading in coffee and caffeine use. Europeans are drinking more coffee than ever. Germans consume over 16 pounds per person each year, and the Swedes lead in consumption with 30 pounds per person per year. The global production of coffee was 7 million tons (14 billion pounds) in 2002 alone, and 2.5 billion pounds of that was consumed in the United States.

Coffee, brewed from the ground coffee bean (*Coffea arabica*), is the major vehicle for caffeine consumption. In this country, more than a half billion cups are consumed daily, with most people drinking two or more cups a day. More than ten pounds of coffee per person are consumed yearly. This food/drug mixture—often combined with sugar and/or milk—is one of the most freely marketed addictive substances in the world.

There are several basic areas of concern, not the least of which focuses on the toxic chemicals used in growing and processing coffee. The oils easily go rancid and the irritating acids contained in the beans themselves offer further hazards. People trying to cut down by drinking decaffeinated coffee could be exposed to even more dangerous chemicals unless they are drinking water-processed decaf and using organically grown beans. This Swiss process uses steam distillation to remove the caffeine, whereas regular decaffeination uses agents such as TCE (trichlorethylene) or methylene chloride, which leave residues in the prepared decaf coffee itself. The last few decades have also seen an increase in the use of pesticides and chemical processing.

In 1946, yearly consumption was twenty pounds per person. Since most children and some adults were not consuming any coffee, many people in 1946 were consuming more than the one-thousand-cup-a-year average. From 1980 to 1990, coffee consumption averaged about ten pounds a year (U.S. Department of Agriculture, annual statistics).

Two trends related to beverage intake are evident: people are developing healthier habits by drinking more light fruit juices, fresh vegetables juices, and water. From 1980 to 1993, the average intake of bottled water increased from 2.4 to 9.2 gallons. Now, the world bottled water market represents an annual volume of 89 billion liters. Sales of bottled water in the United States has continued to experience a huge increase; in 1998 alone, sales grew by 10.1 percent to 3.6 billion gallons. In a 2001 survey, the World Wildlife Fund estimated that people all over the world drink about 89 billion liters of bottled water a year. This is worth about twenty-two million in U.S. dollars. Americans drink about thirteen billion liters of bottled water a year. A 2000 report conducted by Yankelovich Partners of the Rockefeller University discovered that 2.3 eight-ounce servings of the total 6.1 servings of water that are consumed daily per person are bottled water in the United States.

And just as with water intake, coffee consumption is on the rise. Social events increasingly include fashionable coffee beverages such as espresso, cappuccino, and lattes.

Another problem is caffeine's widespread use as an ingredient in so many products, including some soft drinks, energy bars, and many OTC drugs. The problem here is less with the drug itself and more with the amounts consumed and the constant stimulation on which people come to depend many times daily, sometimes unknowingly. One big area of concern here is with children and teenagers, who may consume large amounts of caffeine when drinking soft drinks. Cola naturally contains caffeine, yet many soft drinks have additional amounts that promote an addiction to the drink. Cocoa, which also contains caffeine, has become more popular in the United States.

Another concern is that caffeine is often consumed along with other substances such as nicotine and sugar. Like sugar, caffeine overstimulates the adrenals and then weakens them with persistent or chronic use. A cycle develops where first sugar stimulates and weakens the adrenals, creating fatigue to which we then respond by drinking caffeine to stay awake. In addition, people who overuse caffeine tend to need more tranquilizers and sleeping pills to help them relax or sleep. Caffeine is a lifetime drug for many. We begin at a young age with hot chocolate or chocolate bars, move into colas or other soft drinks, and then add coffee and tea.

Physiologically, caffeine is a central nervous system (CNS) stimulant. It is a member of the class of methylxanthine chemicals/drugs. Xanthines (specifically theophylline) are commonly used in medicine to aid in breathing. Theobromine, another xanthine derivative, is found in cocoa. Methylxanthines are found in many other plants, including the kola nut originally used to make cola drinks.

A dosage of 50 to 100 mg caffeine, the amount in one cup of coffee, will produce a temporary increase in mental clarity and energy levels while simultaneously reducing drowsiness. It also improves muscular-coordinated work activity, such as typing. Through its CNS stimulation, caffeine increases brain activity; however, it also stimulates the cardiovascular system, raising blood pressure and heart rate. It generally speeds up our body by increasing our basal metabolic rate (BMR), which burns more calories. Initially, caffeine may lower blood sugar; however, this can lead to increased hunger or cravings for sweets. After adrenal stimulation, blood sugar rises again. Caffeine also increases respiratory rates, and for people with tight airways, it can open breathing passages (as do the other xanthine drugs). Caffeine is also a diuretic and a mild laxative.

The amount of caffeine needed to produce stimulation increases with regular use, as is typical of all addictive drugs. Larger and more frequent doses are needed to achieve the original effect, and symptoms can develop if we do not get our

SIGNS AND SYMPTOMS OF CAFFEINE INTOXICATION OR ABUSE		
Nervousness	Headache	Increased heart rate
Anxiety	Upset stomach	Irregular heartbeat
Irritability	GI irritation	Elevated blood pressure
Agitation	Heartburn	Increased cholesterol
Tremors	Diarrhea	Nutritional deficiencies
Insomnia	Fatigue	Poor concentration
Depression	Dizziness	Bed wetting

CAFFEINE WITHDRAWAL SYMPTOMS		
Headache	Anxiety	Vomiting
Craving	Nervousness	Cramps
Irritability	Shakiness	Ringing in the ears
Insomnia	Dizziness	Feeling hot and cold
Fatigue	Drowsiness	Tachycardia
Depression	Inability to concentrate	
Apathy	Runny nose	
Constipation	Nausea	

"fix." Eventually, we need the drug to function; without it, fatigue, drowsiness, and headaches can occur.

Unfortunately, most caffeine products do not contain any of the nutrients, such as manganese and copper, needed to support the increased activity that they cause. Also, the diuretic effect of caffeine leads to the urinary loss of many nutrients, which frequently go unreplaced.

Overall, addiction to caffeine is not as bad as addiction to most other drugs. Usually, the slower the tapering of use, the easier the withdrawal. After complete withdrawal and detoxification from caffeine, it is possible to use it in moderation, but care must be taken as it can be re-addicting.

The most common caffeine withdrawal symptom is a throbbing and/or pressure headache, usually located at the temples but occasionally at the back of the head or around the eyes. A vague muscular headache often follows. Of course, caffeine can cure these symptoms; but this is not the answer. Rather, we need to adhere to dietary guidelines and supplements to help with this and other withdrawal problems. It is best to taper off caffeine before going on a cleanse as the withdrawal (mainly headaches) can be very uncomfortable. The Detox Diet works well for this transition.

Coffee is not the only product in our diet that contains caffeine. Of the teas, all black or common teas such as Earl Grey or English Breakfast contain theophylline and theobromine, as do many green teas. Both contain less caffeine than coffee. Tannic acid, a mild irritant to the gastrointestinal mucosa that may reduce absorption of minerals such as manganese, zinc, and copper, can be found in both coffee and tea. Most herbs do not contain caffeine, although maté and guarana are fairly high in caffeine. The kola nut and the cocoa bean also contain caffeine. Ephedra or mahuang is a Chinese herb that gives caffeine-like stimulation. These natural products have been used as stimulants throughout history. There is recent concern with ephedra (and guarana less so) products that are used for energy and weight loss. Many people have problems with nervousness, agitation, fast heart rate, palpitations, and even more dangerous heart issues. There have been some deaths from ephedra use/overuse and deaths, and because of this, there are current legislation attempts to eliminate ephedra stimulants from the public marketplace.

Both extracted and synthesized caffeine may be added to other products. Many common pharmaceutical preparations contain caffeine for its stimulating effects, which counteract the sedating antihistamines, or for its cerebral vasodilating effects used to relieve vascular headaches. Cafergot is a prescription drug containing caffeine and is used for migraines; although caffeine can help reduce headaches, it more commonly causes them.

CAFFEINE DRUGS AVAILABLE OVER THE COUNTER

Stimulants—No-Doz, Vivarin
Weight control—Dexatrim
Pain Relief—Excedrin, Anacin, Vanquish
Menstrual pain relief—Midol
Cold remedies—Dristan

Caffeine, although it is not seriously addicting, is very habit forming. Anyone interested in high-level health should avoid it. Although it may improve short-term performance, it eventually creates long-term depletion.

NEGATIVE EFFECTS OF CAFFEINE

Most of the negative effects of caffeine are not a concern with occasional use, but can occur with regular use of over 100 mg daily. The risks discussed in the following list vary with the level of caffeine intake and individual sensitivity. A total of more than 500 mg of caffeine daily is a high intake, and the total includes all coffee, tea, soft drinks, and drugs. Between 250 and 500 mg might be classified as moderate intake, while less than 250 mg daily would be low. For a long time, the popularity of caffeine outweighed its negative effects. Now the dangers are fairly clear, and it is hard to refute the evidence.

DANIELLA'S CASE STUDY:
J.K., age 30

I am addicted to my daily latte. I have used coffee to pick me up when I am depressed or tired. After drinking it for years I noticed that I didn't get a rush from it anymore. In fact, it made me feel more tired.

Author's note: What J.K. is experiencing is adrenal depletion, which can happen from the overuse or abuse of stimulants. She quit coffee for three months and let her adrenal glands recover. Now she is out of the habit of using coffee and can safely enjoy an occasional cup without feeling drained. She said she also realizes now that she used to experience caffeine-induced anxiety. She is a much calmer and happier person now.

Common negative effects include:

- excess nervousness, irritability, insomnia, "restless legs," dizziness, and subsequent fatigue
- headaches
- "heartburn"
- general anxiety (even panic attacks)
- hyperactivity and bed wetting in children who consume caffeine
- increased stomach hydrochloric acid production (clearly bad for people with existing ulcers or gastritis)
- loss of minerals such as potassium, magnesium, and zinc, and vitamins including the B vitamins, particularly thiamine and vitamin C
- reduced absorption of iron and calcium (especially when caffeine is consumed around mealtime)
- osteoporosis and anemia
- interrupted growth in children and adolescents
- diarrhea
- increased blood pressure and hypertension, especially in atherosclerosis and heart disease
- increased cholesterol and triglyceride blood levels
- heart rhythm disturbances and mild arrhythmias, tachycardia, and palpitations
- increased norepinephrine secretion, which causes some vasoconstriction (although caffeine may have mild vasodilating effects in the heart and body, excess adrenal stimulation may override this)
- increased risk of heart attacks (while results are mixed, it seems reasonable to assume that drinking four to five cups of coffee per day does increase the incidence of myocardial infarctions due to cardiovascular stimulation)
- fibrocystic breast disease (again, results vary, but it is clear that some women experience an increase in size and number of cysts with increased use of caffeine)
- birth defects and spontaneous abortions (Caffeine does cross the placenta and affects the fetus, but the distinct cause of mutagenic effects is not clear. It is wise to limit or completely avoid the use of caffeine during pregnancy and lactation.)
- kidney stones, which can occur as a result of the diuretic and chemical effects

- increased fevers, both as a direct effect and by counteracting the effect of aspirin
- increased incidence of certain cancers including bladder cancer (more frequently due to a combination with nicotine), ovarian cancer, and pancreatic cancer
- prostate enlargement may also be attributed to increased caffeine intake
- adrenal exhaustion/stress/fatigue/hypoglycemia syndrome is tied to caffeine use

While caffeine has the overall effect of increasing blood sugar, stress and sugar intake weaken the adrenal function. Recovery from the resulting fatigue requires rest, stress reduction, and sugar avoidance, and even though caffeine can override this fatigue and restimulate the adrenals temporarily, eventually chronic fatigue, adrenal exhaustion, and subsequent inability to handle any stress or sugar will result. Caffeine will then be of little help.

DETOXIFICATION FROM CAFFEINE

Anyone with a regular caffeine habit should seriously consider discontinuing its use until they can reach a state of occasional enjoyment. If addiction is clear, or in cases of pregnancy, caffeine should be given up completely. Breaking the habit by either tapering off or going "cold turkey" will be easier with a good diet and adrenal support.

Two or three weeks of the Detox Diet can support the transition into a healthier and caffeine-free program. The post-detox diet includes vegetable salads, soups, greens, seaweed, some whole grains, various bean sprouts, and some nuts and seeds, using fruit for snacks. A decreased intake of acid foods such as meat, sugar, and refined flour products is also a good idea, as is avoiding the overuse of baked goods (even whole-grain products), nuts, and seeds. Drinking at least six to eight glasses of filtered water a day and sipping mineral water or herbal teas can help replace the coffee habit. Baking soda or, better, potassium bicarbonate tablets, will not only help make our bodies more alkaline but also reduce some of the withdrawal symptoms.

In addition, vitamin C supplementation helps during withdrawal by supporting the adrenal glands. As a stress-reducer, several grams or more of vitamin C can be taken over the course of the day, preferably in a buffered form, especially with the main alkaline minerals—potassium, calcium, and magnesium—as well as zinc. I also suggest B complex vitamins with extra pantothenic acid (250 mg four times daily), along with 500 mg of vitamin C every two or three hours.

COFFEE CUPFULL
by Bethany Argisle

As one of the most indulged in "food groups," caffeine is not only in coffee, it is in medications, chocolate, and is a body/mind stimulant. When we give no rest to our liver or brain with the other things we add to our cupful, blonde and sweet, all those sugar or aspartame packets, which really create problems in our ability to recover quickly from what might be simple day-to-day stresses.

There is so much to choose from, here in the 21st Century Cupful... So, what desire lurks in my cup? I love the aroma, the ritual of organic coffee—I have eliminated the chemicals used to grow and transport coffee.

When Elson took me for a visit to Andrew Weil's home many years ago, I was fascinated by a story he told me about the power of coffee as a drug in Amazonian cultures, where it was mixed into a strong brew in villages, along with cayenne pepper to make a drug that would send the village into a frenzy of healing, of settling debts, of facing betrayals. The purpose of this concoction was to heal the village so it could go on hunting and being familial for its basic survival, and this was done on a regular basis in order to create a continuum of life. It seems the village shaman knew how powerful this drug really is when used in cultural context.

We have our stimulants, we have liver replacements, we have pre-packaged and speedy foods, and all of these things together place constant stresses on a body that is already dealing with environmental pollution.

Sure, I drink coffee, I began when I was a young teen and remember how my mother used to let me have an occasional "grown-up" cup, which was half milk with tons of sugar—very yum—and to this day I get that same feeling. Of course I try to keep it down to what I drink at home and an occasional exotic coffee when I am on the road.

I agree with Dr. Haas—if you can take a break from coffee at least ten days, twice a year, then you are the master or mistress of your own liver, your eyes, your digestion. Is it easy? No way! Yet, I did it. That is why I attended my last detox group with Dr. Haas and why Dr. Gabriel Cousens put me on two adrenal burnout healings at his juice and yoga retreats.

If you want to continue your coffee cups, it is important to know exactly what you are doing to your health. Yes, several "healers" have given me coffee substitutes and alternatives, most all of which make me want another cup of coffee. I believe taking a break is a good health choice on a regular basis.

CAFFEINE LEVELS* IN COMMON SUBSTANCES**

Coffee and Other Drinks/6 oz cup	Amount of Caffeine (mg)
Drip	120–150
Percolated	80–110
Instant	60–70
Decaf	3–10
Espresso (1 oz shot)	75
Caffe Latte	70
Cappuccino	70
Caffe Mocha	80
Black tea	50–60
Earl Grey	50
English Breakfast	50
Green tea	30–40
Jasmine	20
Cocoa	10–30
Chocolate milk	10–15
Cocoa (dry, 1 oz)	40–50
Chocolate (dry, 1 oz)	5–10

Soft drink/12 oz serving	
Colas	30–65
Mountain Dew	50

OTC Medicines	
No-Doz	100
Vivarin	200
Dexatrim	200
Dietac	200
Cafergot	100
Excedrin	65
Fiorinal	40
Anacin	30
Vanquish	35
Midol	30

* These caffeine levels and caffeine equivalents may depend on length of brewing time or amount of product used. The levels given are approximate.
** Information gathered and integrated from at least six different sources.

During average coffee use, we need to be careful to replenish depleted nutrients including thiamine (B$_1$), riboflavin (B$_2$), pyridoxine (B$_6$), vitamin C, potassium, magnesium, and, to a lesser degree, zinc, iron, calcium, and the trace minerals. Additional amino acids can help balance our energy level during use of or withdrawal from caffeine. Water intake and additional fiber will support bowel function, which frequently slows down during caffeine withdrawal.

Spreading the detoxification program over a week or two and reducing caffeine intake to none will help avoid significant headaches. Lower caffeine intake by drinking grain-coffee blends, diluted or smaller amounts of regular coffee, or decaffeinated coffee (water processed). Another approach is to first substitute black tea, which has less caffeine than coffee, and which can be tapered more easily.

If headaches occur, mild pain relievers can be used for a few days, but avoid taking them over a longer period of time. Increased water intake, vitamin C and mineral support, an alkaline diet, and white willow bark herb tablets, which contain a natural salicylate, should ease these withdrawal symptoms.

There are a number of herbal teas to use in place of coffee that can be both stimulating and refreshing. The roasted herbal roots, including barley, chicory, and dandelion, are most popular. Grain "coffees," such as Barley Coffee, Cafix, Inka, Postum, Pero, Rombouts, Raja's Cup, and Wilson's Heritage, are also favored among former coffee drinkers, while ginseng root tea is preferred by some. Teechino is a tasty and popular grain beverage that helps some coffee users transition to this healthier drink. Herbal teas made from lemon grass, peppermint, ginger root, red clover, and comfrey are very nourishing, and do not have the depleting side effects. The algaes can also be energizing in place of caffeine.

If we do like a cup of coffee or caffeinated tea a day, it might be best to drink it in the mid- to late afternoon, which is different from what most people do, using caffeine as their wake-up call and for energy through the day. The afternoon cup best fits our body's natural cycle, avoiding the high-adrenal morning and late pre-sleep hours. Those who cannot relax or sleep well after using caffeine should consider avoiding it altogether.

The pleasures of coffee and tea drinking are as much a cultural phenomenon as they are a taste preference. Remember, habits are developed, not inherent, and anything we learn, we can also unlearn or relearn.

Use the lower ranges of nutrients in the following table for general support and the higher levels for detoxification. The amounts shown are daily totals and should be divided into two or three supplementations during the day.

HERBAL CAFFEINE SUBSTITUTES

Roasted barley	Rombouts	Ginseng root
Chicory root	Rostaroma	Ginger root
Dandelion root	Wilson's Heritage	Comfrey leaf
Teechin	Cafix	Lemon grass
Postum	Miso broth	Red clover
Pero	Duran	Comfrey leaf
Pioneer	Peppermint	

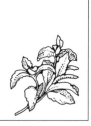

CAFFEINE SUPPORT AND DETOX NUTRIENT PROGRAM

Water	2½–3 qt	Calcium	800–1,000 mg
Fiber	15–20 g	Chromium	200–400 mcg
Vitamin A	5,000–10,000 IU	Copper	2–3 mg
Mixed carotenoids	15,000–30,000 IU	Iodine	150 mcg
Vitamin D	400 IU	Iron*	
Vitamin E	400–800 IU	men	0–15 mg
Vitamin K	300 mcg	women	15–30 mg
Thiamine (B_1)	75–150 mg	Magnesium	500–800 mg
Riboflavin (B_2)	50–100 mg	Manganese	5–10 mg
Niacinamide (B_3)	50–100 mg	Molybdenum	300–500 mcg
Niacin (B_3)	50–100 mg	Potassium	300–600 mg
Pantothenic acid (B_5)	500–1,000 mg	Silicon	50–100 mg
Pyridoxine (B_6)	50–100 mg	Selenium	200–300 mcg
Pyridoxal-5-phosphate	25–50 mg	Zinc	30–60 mg
Cobalamin (B_{12})	100–200 mcg	Adrenal	50–150 mg
Folic acid	400–800 mcg	L-amino acids	500–1,500 mg
Biotin	300 mcg	Potassium bicarbonate**	600–1,000 mg
Vitamin C	2–6 g	Herbal teas	3 cups daily
Bioflavonoids	250–500 mg	Blue-green algae	500–2,000 mg

* Level would depend on lab values; otherwise, use only 10 mg/day maximum.
** Can use Alka-Seltzer Effervescent Antacid, one tablet 2 to 3 times daily. Antacids used excessively or with meals may interfere with proper digestion.

CAFFEINE DETOX SUMMARY

1. If you take in more than 500 mg a day of caffeine, consider taking a break from it, and clearing your body of caffeine. If you are pregnant and have high caffeine intake detox under the guidance of a health-care practitioner.

2. After that, avoid the daily use of caffeine. For most people, it can still be tolerated and enjoyed as long as it does not become a daily habit.

3. Consider the Detox Diet or a general alkaline diet consisting mainly of vegetables, both steamed and as salads, fruits, plus some whole grains, and some protein, such as a few nuts or seeds, or a little fish or poultry if you feel it's needed.

4. Drink at least 6 to 8 glasses of water daily or more, especially if you exercise and sweat.

5. Keep fiber intake high to help clear the colon and support detoxification.

6. Supplement your nutrition with vitamins and minerals as outlined.

7. If headaches occur, as they commonly do in the first few days of detox, increase your intake of water, vitamin C, and minerals, and use white willow bark herb to ease headaches and withdrawal.

8. Other herbs, particularly as teas, can be taken to support the body or as coffee substitutes.

CHAPTER ELEVEN

Drug Detoxification

Drug detoxification involves two main processes—changing our abusive habits (not using the drugs) and releasing the drug residues from our bodies and our lives.

We are a drug culture, and Western medicine is likewise a drug-oriented system. We consume billions of pills yearly and spend many billions of dollars buying them. These figures do not even begin to include the everyday use of caffeine, alcohol, and nicotine. There are really no stereotypical drug addicts anymore. Affluent or poor people, anyone under pressure or with unmet psychological needs can end up with this problem. Substance abuse is an individual, family, and worldwide problem that can affect young and old, men and women. And in truth, most people in modern Western cultures are addicted to one or more substances/drugs, sugar and caffeine being the most common.

It is important to understand the relationship between states of being, symptoms, and our use of drugs. In other words, if we view a symptom as problematic, we want to correct it with drugs. Although for immediate relief this may seem practical, it is theoretically shortsighted and shows a complete misunderstanding of human body design. In actuality, drug use and drug therapy rarely fix anything. Our symptoms serve as a warning sign of some bigger problem for which we must determine the cause. Symptoms are not the real problem, but rather are the results of deeper processes and causes. They are also not errors on the part of our body since our body rarely errs; rather, our body responds to the way we treat it. To correct aggravating symptoms, we must correct our internal imbalances and usually alter our lives. It is very important not to devitalize our body in any way if we can possibly avoid it. Since much habitual drug use is part of a syndrome of self-destruction, the first step for many people is to learn to care for and love themselves again, reinforcing their desire to live.

Pharmaceutical prescriptions and most over-the-counter (OTC) drugs are designed to help us feel better, yet they are too often used to treat problems resulting from abusive or misguided habits. This may aggravate the original problem or cause side effects. The promotion of addictions (which both support and drain our economy) begins with an emphasis on sugar. In fact, the use of sugar is so pervasive in our culture that it is difficult to find prepared or packaged foods that do not contain sugar or other sweeteners. Our habitual sweet tooth progresses to addictive usage of caffeine, nicotine, alcohol, and foods such as wheat, refined foods, and milk products. Later, the coffee break (combined with sugary snacks or coffee sweeteners) becomes a reward— a refueling rest stop during the workday. Caffeine and sugar stimulate us to work more. Nervousness and hyperactivity are often associated with productivity, although they are really not comparable to steady, healthful energy. Trying to perpetuate that productivity through the use of artificial stimulants eventually leads to reduced capacity, time lost from work, wasted money, and increased illness. Our behavior regarding foods, particularly sweet ones, is conditioned very early and is very difficult to change.

All drugs have some toxicity. Most have both physiological and psychological actions and addictive potential that result in accumulated toxicity and withdrawal symptoms when we try to give them up. **Before going through any drug or chemical detoxification, it is wise to prepare for it.** This is important both physically and psychologically, and it is definitely helpful to have a physician or other health-care provider, therapist or counselor, family member or good friend for support. The withdrawal phase poses the most difficulties and can last from a day or two to a week or more. It is often hard to differentiate the physical sensations from the underlying psychological involvement. The withdrawal phase itself is part of the drug addiction cycle; in other words, the worse the withdrawal, the more likely we are to continue to use the chemical to prevent those symptoms. A psychological dependency easily develops from the physical dependency.

After the initial withdrawal, where we detoxify through the release of stored chemicals from the body, we need willpower and commitment to keep the particular substance out of our life. We also need to work on new behavior patterns, such as avoiding exposure to the people and places associated with our previous problem until we develop new habits. Those new habits need to be strong enough so that we can easily say no when we are exposed to the substance again. Behavior modification therapy can be very helpful.

Characteristics of addiction include needing the drug to function, needing it in ever higher doses, needing it more frequently, feeling sick when a dose is missed, and/or having a history of abuse or addiction. The most useful approach to dealing with drug addiction begins with admitting that there is a problem. We must then combine our desire and willpower to accomplish this difficult task—detox and recovery—and there are many support programs and government resources to help (see page xxx). This decision often arises during illness or crisis rather than as a true desire to be healthy. Nonetheless, whatever gets us there is just fine, as long as we have the determination to follow through and stay on the path.

A well-balanced diet and a good nutritional supplement program are essential to an effective plan, as is some psychological support. During the transition, either a cleansing diet or a fast is helpful to enhance purification and lessen the severity and length of withdrawal. I have seen people make dramatic lifestyle changes with only a week-long cleanse. Their new sense of empowerment helps them to clarify their goals while reinforcing their willpower.

The Detox Diet program, which focuses primarily on steamed vegetables with some additional fruit and grains, allows a smooth transition with minimal withdrawal. It works to increase alkalinity and reduce acidity, which supports natural detoxification. Cravings and withdrawal intensify with an acid state generated by meats, milk products, and refined flours and sugars. A general diet that emphasizes fruits and vegetables, juices and soups, or even water can be used temporarily, as these are all alkaline-forming.

I do not suggest withdrawing or detoxifying from drugs during illness or either right before or after surgery, although sometimes it is unavoidable. However, during pregnancy (ideally before pregnancy), it is important to clear all unnecessary drugs including OTC drugs, alcohol, nicotine, and caffeine. In all cases, we must be careful when withdrawing from these substances, although usually the basic daily habits can be tapered off and eliminated over the course of a few days. Since fetal stability is vitally important, it would be wise to have medical supervision during any form of detoxification during pregnancy.

Supplemental nutrients also support the system during drug elimination. Vitamin C and the other antioxidants—vitamins A and E, zinc and selenium, L-cysteine and other amino acids—are particularly important, in addition to a basic vitamin and mineral supplement. Glutathione, which is formed from L-cysteine in the body, acts in detoxification enzymes and helps decrease the toxicity of most drugs and chemicals.

A nutritional supplement approach to drug detoxification includes the B vitamins, minerals, a high amount of vitamin C, antioxidants, and the L-amino acids. These are more efficient when combined with a food diet than with fasting, and thus the alkaline, fruit- and vegetable-based diet is a better complement to any high nutrient intake. With a more liquid diet, Minimize your intake of supplements and add more vitamin C, some minerals, and an antioxidant formula, along with herbs and chlorophyll or algae products.

Herbal therapies can also be helpful. Goldenseal root powder is probably the most important herb as it not only stimulates the liver to better perform its detox function but also helps clear toxicity with its alkaloids. Take one large or two small capsules twice daily before meals for one or two weeks. Milk thistle, specifically *Silybum marianum*, also protects the liver from toxins and supports the detoxification process. Other helpful herbs during drug detoxification are those that work as laxatives, diuretics, and blood or lymph cleansers (see page 223 for a list of detoxifying herbs). Valerian root and other tranquilizing herbs may also lessen excitatory withdrawal symptoms such as anxiety or insomnia. Chlorophyll, taken as tablets or liquid, has a mildly purifying and rejuvenating quality.

PHARMACEUTICALS—PRESCRIPTION AND OTC DRUGS

Any prescription or OTC drug can be toxic, especially when used too much or for too long. Aspirin, anti-inflammatory and pain-relieving drugs, tranquilizers, and anti-depressants are all in common use and are all similarly toxic, especially to the gastrointestinal tract. The same is true for antibiotics, used millions of times a day across the country to treat many kinds of apparently infectious illnesses, which natural medicine thinkers believe are the body's attempts to cleanse itself and heal by releasing mucus debris, creating fevers, and inflaming membranes. Regular use/overuse of these incredibly valuable real infection treatments also cause imbalances, allergic reactions, and digestive tract disturbances. Keeping ourselves healthy and clear is the prime way to stay away from using these strong drug therapies.

In other words, **the key to preventing the need to detoxify from drugs is to avoid their use in the first place.** Many people are turning from Western medicine to alternative therapies and remedies as better preparation and knowledge have improved their efficacy. When used correctly, they support our body's natural healing powers and correct imbalances. Consult with a knowledgeable practitioner or information source for appropriate guidance, as herbs and other natural remedies (as well as homeopathy) can produce occasional side effects as well. Acupuncture, osteopathic and chiropractic therapies, massage, and other body work can stimulate elimination and natural healing during detoxification periods.

Although OTC products are usually less toxic than pharmaceuticals, they are also more frequently abused as they can be readily obtained and are less expensive than most prescription drugs. Many symptoms are commonly treated with specific OTC drugs, seen in the following chart.

COMMON OTC DRUGS	
Symptoms	**Drugs**
Headache	Aspirin, acetaminophen, ibuprofen
Fatigue	Caffeine, nicotine, No-Doz
Insomnia	Tranquilizers, antihistamines
Colds, flus	Antihistamines, decongestants
Allergies	Laxatives, lubricants
Constipation	Kaopectate, fibers
Diarrhea	Antacids, Pepto-Bismol, Alka-Seltzer
Indigestion	Stimulants, such as Ephedra and Phertenmine
Excess weight	

Even at low potencies, many of these OTC drugs can create physical dependency. This is true especially when there is a chronic problem that requires long-term usage or when there are withdrawal or rebound symptoms. If problems persist we should consult our health-care practitioner to help us determine the underlying cause and work to correct that rather than continue to treat the symptoms alone. If stress and worry are the cause of insomnia or if poor food choices or meal times lead to our gastrointestinal symptoms, we need to make some lifestyle changes. If the symptoms persist, herbs or homeopathy are more gentle remedies.

Aspirin and caffeine are at the top of the OTC drug problems list. (Caffeine is discussed thoroughly in Chapter 10.) Aspirin, a valuable medicine in common use for many decades, is on the decline due to GI irritation and other concerns. Acetaminophen (Tylenol), ibuprofen (Advil, Motrin), and other anti-inflammatory medications (NSAIDs—Non-Steroidal Anti-Inflammatory Drugs) have reduced the overall intake of aspirin. However, they come with their own health risks. Americans take on the average 24 doses of NSAIDs per person per year, and since most don't take this, that's a lot in those using these drugs. This class of medications irritates the intestinal lining, which leads to internal bleeding and ulcers in many cases. Over 100,000 people are hospitalized in the United States. each year due to intestinal bleeding from NSAID use. Often those hospitalized use moderate doses. Many people use these medications at the first sign of swelling or discomfort, but they should only be used when necessary and after other more natural therapies are used. This includes massage and chiropractic for musculoskeletal pain, relaxation, rest, and detox for headaches, and herbal and nutritional products. *Detox helps many aches and pains, so follow this book, and you won't need to call me in the morning.*

Acetylsalicylic acid (aspirin), derived from coal tar, has over fifty million regular users in this country consuming 20,000 tons of aspirin and 225 tablets per person per year in the United States. Aspirin formulas often contain caffeine and act as anti-inflammatory agents. Aspirin works to reduce fevers (which, if left alone, are natural healers) and tends to work better than its counterpart acetaminophen. Both drugs are now in common use as people experience more pain and more degenerative conditions, such as cardiovascular disease. Low doses of aspirin have been found to reduce blood clotting effects and are commonly taken to reduce heart attack and stroke risk as one baby aspirin (81 mg) a day. (The typical aspirin tablet for adults is 325 mg, whereby two to three of those are taken to relieve the pain of arthritis, for example.)

The key to eliminating anti-inflammatory drugs is to eliminate the pain for which they are taken. Stronger pain drugs include the anti-inflammatory medicines like ibuprofen and the new ones Vioxx and Celebrex; most of these drugs have side effects, especially in the gastrointestinal tract. Pain problems are frequently treated with even stronger prescription narcotics, such as codeine (aspirin or acetaminophen with codeine is very commonly used), hydrocodone (Vicodin), propoxyphene (Darvon), or even Demerol or morphine. All of these narcotic drugs are much more addictive and thus more difficult to stop using; however, they are tolerated better by some people than other medicines.

TRANSITION FROM DRUGS TO NATURAL THERAPIES

I began studying and working with natural medicines only after I learned about and was prescribing pharmaceutical drugs. Upon investigation, I became aware that many of the drugs I was prescribing had their basis or origin in plants. Some examples are Valium from valerian root, Ipecac from ipecaquana root, and digitalis from the foxglove plant. Scientists studied the active plant ingredients and then synthesized like molecules and stronger variations of those phytochemicals.

Well, I think we lost something in the transition, namely, the safety and general positive effects with minimal side effects. We gained something also—power and speed.

These drugs have greater, though sometimes more limited, effects, and of course, they usually have side effects and potential toxicity.

Over the last three decades, I have taken a back-to-nature approach. That means living more closely to and with greater reverence for nature, and thus paying closer attention to how I live. I eat more wholesomely and exercise and relax outdoors as often as possible. I have come to the awareness that my body is a part of nature, not separate from her. After more than twenty-five years of finely tuning this awareness, I have learned to sense the subtlest adverse changes in my body. Since they are more subtle and less symptomatic, I can correct them with less invasive and safer therapies, specifically dietary changes, nutritional supplements, herbal and homeopathic remedies, body work, rest and quiet, and hands-on therapies.

I encourage you to try a natural remedy the next time you experience a problem, unless of course, you believe your condition to be serious or dangerous. Some common ailments with examples of natural therapies are as follows:

NATURAL THERAPIES FOR COMMON PROBLEMS

- **Fatigue**—adequate rest and good sleep, breathing and meditation, massage, nutritional supplements, along with ginseng and other herbs
- **Insomnia**—exercise, calcium and magnesium, valerian root and other herbs, melatonin, and L-tryptophan (or 5-HTP)
- **Headache**—rest, water, detox, walk on the beach, colon cleanse, white willowbark
- **Colds or Flu**—sleep, fluids, vitamins C and A, echinacea, goldenseal root, or olive leaf
- **Constipation**—water, fiber, fruits and vegetables, abdominal massage, laxative herbs
- **Indigestion**—water and herb teas like peppermint, chamomile or licorice root, aloe vera juice, activated charcoal (for gas), assess for parasites and other abnormal microbes
- **Allergies**—water, detox and juicing, vitamin C, quercetin, and herbs like nettle

One of the most exciting and rewarding aspects of my "natural-first" medical practice is the positive results my patients experience with minimal or no side effects. Over the years, they've discovered for themselves that eating well and exercising regularly removes the need to even consider taking drugs because they don't get sick! (Of course, if someone is acutely ill and/or in danger medically, I will use the quicker and stronger medications, and then later work to transition them to a more natural therapy.) **My philosophy of practice is simple—lifestyle first, natural therapies next, and drugs last.**

Please realize that all treatments, be they dietary changes, nutritional supplements and herbs, or drugs, are an experiment, or more accurately, an *experience*. Until you try them yourself, you cannot really know their exact effect upon your symptoms, disease, or health. To properly assess this personal experiment, be patient and be aware of and attentive to changes that occur. Initially, you may experience some adverse or unusual side effects, as in cleansing or healing reactions, but these should pass relatively quickly. (This is discussed more thoroughly in Chapters 2 and 3.)

More commonly, and importantly, there are many positive side effects (I call them "side benefits" instead) and healthful rewards to using natural therapies. Patients often report feeling clear headed, physically energized, spiritually rejuvenated, and ready to set new goals and make new commitments. They look and feel younger, and have a vital, new sense of self with a more expansive and connected understanding. The key is to give nature a chance. After all, you didn't accumulate the excess weight, poor digestion, ill health, or addictive habits overnight.

OTHER DRUGS—STREET AND RECREATIONAL

Street or "recreational" narcotics are also a major social (and health) problem and generally pose a greater, though not insurmountable, challenge to detoxification. These include opium, methadone, heroin, and "crack." Heroin alone has over half a million addicted users. The drug creates a mix of euphoria and depression and also reduces the appetite and libido; and in more extreme situations, basic life needs become less important than the users' lives, which become focused upon obtaining and ingesting the drug. There are many individuals who are in various stages of recovery from drugs, including alcohol and narcotics, and still others in methadone support centers. Dealing with drug dependence has many levels of cause and cure—physical, mental, emotional, and spiritual. Commitment to the path is a healthy philosophy in this regard.

In our medical system, there are many prescription pill habits begun and continued every year. Sleeping pills, tranquilizers, and antidepressants are all frequently prescribed and used to handle life's frustrations and challenges. In many instances, the problem is the poor diet and stress, and the use of the stimulant and sedative daily drugs (the SNACCs) as reviewed in this book; then, changing these lifestyle patterns may help alleviate the mood and energy dysfunctions that we just end up treating and fighting with the basic results of life. Valium was once the number one choice for stressed out and anxious people (starting with unhappy housewives). Now, newer drugs such as Ativan, Xanax, and Buspar are gaining in popularity as they offer tranquilization and sedation of life's stresses. (Barbiturates used to be the main sedative but are now more frequently found on the street.) These drugs affect anxiety by depressing our nervous system in a way somewhat like alcohol. Use the principles and protocol described in the Alcohol chapter (Chapter 9) if these drugs are being taken.

Stimulants such as amphetamines and cocaine can cause dramatic fluctuations in energy. They excite the nervous system and promote euphoria or irritability but result in a loss of appetite, hypersensitivity, and insomnia, usually followed by fatigue and depression. The amphetamine stimulants like Dexedrine and Desoxyn, even though less popular than in prior years, still remain a problem for some. As with the narcotics, amphetamine withdrawal and detoxification often require professional assistance, although some people manage it on their own. The stimulant drugs in general are more deadly than others as they stress and damage the body (cocaine and amphetamines are known for this), so it is very important to eliminate them if we want to live healthfully.

Marijuana (*Cannabis sativa* and *indica*) has become the second most common drug used in the world after alcohol (and not counting caffeine and sugar). And now with its medical effects and potential help in some symptomatic situations (nausea and headaches, for example) as well as health conditions (pain from cancer and other diseases, and loss of appetite from AIDS), it has become a challenge to know how to proceed on a state and national level. Furthermore, we have the related, non-psychoactive hemp plant, which has more useful functions in textiles (clothing), fuels, rope, paper, and more, which would be a great resource for us tree-lovers. An honest reassessment of both medical marijuana and industrial hemp is long overdue.

Smoking marijuana can be a problematic drug habit also, and like other substances, we need to find that healthy and non-dependent relationship. When it's used daily to feel high instead of dealing with emotions and life, it can be destructive. Overall, we can generally say that the least drugs we use, the better.

Again, if you have an active drug problem, stopping totally can be dangerous. You may need a slower transition or guidance and support. *Going "cold turkey" from sedatives, stimulants, and narcotics can have very serious consequences, including seizures.* There are many doctors and facilities, such as hospital detox centers, available to help us deal with drug problems. A further discussion of and specific treatments for drug abuse are beyond the scope of this book. Many of the suggestions in this text, specifically the Detox Diet and Nutritional Supplement guidelines, however, can be very useful in the process of detoxifying from such destructive habits. Also the Niacin-Sauna Therapy, as described on page 105, can be used to support drug detoxification.

The following program is intended as a supplement to a medical drug detoxification program and as support during necessary drug use. The ranges given allow for varying needs. During initial withdrawal, the higher levels should be used, with mid-range levels used during the three to six weeks directly following initial withdrawal. Lower ranges may provide basic support during general drug use.

DRUG DETOXIFICATION NUTRIENT PROGRAM

Water	2–3½ qt	Bioflavonoids	250–500 mg
Fiber	20–40 g	Quercetin	250–600 mg
Vitamin A	5,000–10,000 IU	Calcium	650–1,200 mg+
Mixed carotenoids	20,000–40,000 IU	Chromium	200–500 mcg
Vitamin D	200–400 IU	Copper	2–3 mg
Vitamin E	200–800 IU	Iodine	150 mcg
Vitamin K	300 mcg	Iron	10–20 mg**
Thiamine (B$_1$)	25–100 mg	Magnesium	400–800 mg+
Riboflavin (B$_2$)	25–100 mg	Manganese	5–10 mg
Niacinamide (B$_3$)	50–100 mg	Molybdenum	150–300 mcg
Niacin (B$_3$)	50–1,000 mg*	Potassium	100–500 mg
Pantothenic acid (B$_5$)	250–1,000 mg	Selenium	200–300 mcg
Pyridoxine (B$_6$)	25–100 mg	Silicon	50–150 mg
Pyridoxal-5-phosphate	25–50 mg	Vanadium	200–400 mcg
Cobalamin (B$_{12}$)	100–250 mcg	Zinc	30–60 mg
Folic acid	800 mcg	L-amino acids	1,000–1,500 mg
Biotin	300 mcg	L-cysteine	250–500 mg
Choline	500–1,000 mg	L-glutamine	250–1,000 mg
Inositol	500–1,000 mg	Essential fatty acids	2–4 capsules
Vitamin C	2–10 g	Flaxseed oil	2–4 teaspoons
		Goldenseal root	3–6 capsules

* Increase dosage slowly.
** As needed if low.
+ Higher amounts are needed for hyperactive withdrawal states, aches, or cravings.

DRUG DETOX SUMMARY

1. Drink plenty of water and consider the alkalinizing Detox Diet to help you transition from your habit.
2. If you are a heavy drug user, use the assistance of a health care practitioner or a clinic to support your detox. Going "cold turkey" from sedatives, stimulants, and narcotics can have very serious consequences, including seizures.
3. If you are pregnant, use medical supervision to stop using drugs. Acupuncture has a particularly good reputation for helping moms detox and supporting full-term, healthy babies.
4. Reduce stress in your life. Enhance your coping strategies and support systems.
5. Use psychological supports that fit your value system: counseling, biofeedback, DA (Drugs Anonymous), or behavior modification.
6. Use supplemental nutrients to support your body during detox. Include regular vitamin C, B vitamins, and most minerals, particularly calcium and magnesium for their calming effects.
7. Try herbal therapies to ease the detox process—white willow bark for pains, valerian root and others for anxiety and insomnia. If these are not strong enough, prescription medications can be used temporarily to help ease withdrawal.
8. Consider the use of acupuncture and Chinese herbal therapy to ease the body through its transition.
9. Instead of reaching outwardly for a substance or other crutch, practice breathing and relaxation will follow.

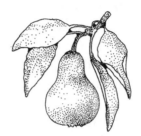

CHAPTER TWELVE

Nontoxic Living

◆

Now that we've talked about cleaning up our diet and our body, how do we decrease toxicity in our home? Here are some ideas for effective cleaning supplies, well-made kitchen tools, and safe drinking water.

THE "NEW" OLD WAY OF CLEANING

We remember our grandmothers hanging the laundry out to dry on the line rather than using the electrical dryer. She saved money and electricity this way, got a lot of exercise, and her sheets smelled like heaven. Now we have a chemical spray or solution for every cleaning need to make it easier and faster. However, the environment and our bodies become unhealthier with every use, and we end up creating new chemical compounds when numerous chemicals are mixed. We don't know how these new chemicals will affect us in the future or how much our bodies are suffering now because of our exposure to them. In the long run, the people and the environment lose and the chemical companies win (only, however, if we consider mere money as winning).

The good news is that we are not dependant on these products. In fact, there are many natural solutions for good cleaning. There are natural and nontoxic ways to get the same results you would achieve with standard chemical cleaning products. For example, most people think of Drano when their sinks become clogged, but it is extremely toxic to your body, the pipes, and to the environment. Instead you could use a snake (a long piece of equipment) to clean out your drain. You may be surprised at how effective it is, and you'll save money in the long run. Also vinegar and baking soda poured in equal parts down the drain, followed by a plunger, will unclog a slow-draining sink or tub in many cases.

Another example of nontoxic cleaning alterative is for your microwave, when it has food odors that won't go away. Rather than use harsh cleaning sprays, just wipe it out with lemon juice mixed with water to freshen it up. Squeeze half a lemon in a cup of water. The lemon acids help cut grease as well.

Avoid antibacterial soaps and cleansers, which are harsh and add to the problem of antibiotic-resistant organisms. Some chemicals we use daily in our homes are not all that toxic on their own, but once they come in contact with other chemicals they turn into toxic chemical compounds. For example, when chlorine bleach combines with ammonia it forms a deadly gas. There are so many effective natural cleaning products available today that there is no reason to continue using toxic formulas (see the resources that follow and at the back of the book).

IN THE KITCHEN

With a few simple changes in kitchen equipment you will be able to reduce contact with synthetic materials and considerably reduce your chemical exposure overall. Here are some specific ideas:

- Avoid plastic Tupperware and use glass bowls such as those from Crate and Barrel, or use ceramics instead of plastics. When food is heated in plastics some of the plastic material ends up in the food, especially if the food contains acids (such as tomatoes or lemons.) Glass does not leach anything into the food and is a much safer choice. Also, be sure that any ceramic you use for preparing or serving food is nontoxic. Some heirloom and imported ceramics may not be food-safe as they may contain lead, arsenic, and other metals.

- Kitchen tools, such as pots and pans that we use daily, can make a big difference in our toxic load. Avoid non-clad aluminum and use only aluminum coated with stainless steel such as All-Clad cookware, stainless steel pans such as Revere Ware, or cast iron skillets. If you have nonstick pots or pans, be sure to use high-temp rated plastic utensils so you don't scrape the non-stick coating (such as Teflon). Once the cookware has been scratched, it will begin to peel and bits of it end up in the food cooked on that surface. Avoiding Teflon pans is really best.

- Pressure cookers allow you to cook nutritious whole foods (such as cooking beans) quickly and efficiently. The Kuhn Rikon pressure cooker is my favorite. For low-fat cooking, the bamboo steamer is the ultimate tool. Also having a blender for smoothies, a small food processor for grinding flaxseed, nuts, and herbs, and a mortar and pestle to grind spices, which releases their natural oils, gives you more freedom in preparing healthy foods.

- A garlic press is a must if you love fresh garlic. The Zyliss Susi garlic press works exceptionally well. Also the rubber garlic tubes sold in kitchen stores work well to remove the garlic skin. A high-quality rubber spatula will help you get that last drop out of jars. OXO makes high-temperature resistance spatulas. A tea ball allows you to sample a wider variety of teas as so many come in loose form rather than in bags. Having a few different cutting boards is a good idea, one for meats and one for produce. Rinse the produce board regularly and pour boiling water over the meat board or run it through the dishwasher frequently.

CLEAN UP YOUR AREA
by Bethany Argisle

Detox your kitchen, your cupboards, and refrigerator; not just your body, but your entire food attitude.

Are you one who thinks their food is grown in the supermarket and harvested from shelves and stored in your refrigerator? I prefer food that grows, is alive, and is made of the seasons and of the elements.

What's the oldest, moldiest food in your kitchen? And, is anything really alive in you, in your refrigerator, in your cupboards, and in all that packaging? Keep dates on your containers, because identification may not be possible later—what with ice burn, and the success of molds, and aliens made out of leftovers.

Replace baking soda in the refrigerator at least every three months. Circulate those ice cubes, and wash your refrigerator handle with a natural cleaning product for a healthy food storage area.

WATER PURIFICATION

Clean water is our most basic need. You can filter water at your kitchen tap with either a reverse osmosis or a solid-carbon activated charcoal filter and use it for all of your drinking water, cooking, and for your pets as well.

The European bottled waters such as Perrier and Evian, and American waters, Trinity, or Ice Age, are high-quality clean waters. The regulations for bottling water in Europe are very strict, and the water is tested at the source as it is being bottled each hour for contamination. Also, I like the sparkling waters like Calistoga, Crystal Geyser, and Talking Rain, which have a little natural flavoring added such as berry, lime, lemon, or orange. The carbonated waters are generally bubbly because of the addition of CO_2, which is safe and easy for our bodies to handle. However, sugared sodas, such as colas, are carbonated with phosphoric acid, and excess phosphorous can have negative health effects. Phosphorous reduces calcium absorption into the bone and contributes to bone loss, which can lead to osteoporosis.

The bottled waters mentioned do not contain anything but pure water, electrolytes, and possible CO_2 or natural fruit flavors. They contain no calories and are tasty soda alternatives. See *The Staying Healthy Shopper's Guide* for more information on water.

Keep bubbly water on hand and add pomegranate or orange juice to make a festive drink or use the sparkling water in place of tonic water, which has a surprising amount of sugar in it.

CHEMICAL-FREE CLOTHING

There are many companies nowadays that promote natural fibers and organic materials. One popular one is Patagonia (www.patagonia.com). This famous outdoor-wear maker has an entire line of organic cotton clothing. Cotton is one of the most heavily treated (with insecticides) crops in the United States. Organic cotton is especially important for those with sensitive skin, babies, and the elderly.

Some interesting facts from Patagonia's website:

- You are what you choose. Organic clothing, like organic food, is vital to protecting the health of our farmlands, our waterways, our environment, and ultimately ourselves. The choices you make when you buy food and clothing affect us all.

- Conventional cotton farming accounts for 25 percent of the world's insecticide use. And the pesticides used on cotton are some of the most toxic.

- At least 107 active ingredients in pesticides are carcinogenic.

- Farming pesticides already contaminate groundwater in 32 states and half of the U.S. population relies on groundwater for drinking.

- Children are at greater risk for pesticide-related health problems and millions of U.S. children already receive their lifetime dose of some carcinogenic pesticides by age 5.

Natural fibers such as hemp and linen are made into fabrics and clothing and are available on the Internet or in stores. These fabrics are generally made from plants that are organically grown and untreated with chemicals.

NATURAL CLEANING PRODUCTS

As mentioned, this is an important area for all of us who live on planet Earth to consider, since we all contribute to pollution by the cleaning and laundering choices we make in our home. There are many companies, and more entering this area of commerce, that are conscientious and caring about the quality of products they sell. Here are a few of those companies.

Caldrea (www.caldrea.com)—Caldrea has a full line of natural cleaners that are not only effective but are scented with essential oils, which make you feel like you're at a spa when you're cleaning. The product line includes countertop cleansers, toilet cleaner, wood furniture cleaner, window/glass cleaner, all-purpose cleaners, liquid dish soap, and scented linen water. They come in Jasmine-Lily and Lavender-Pine scents and are sold in kitchen stores, gift shops, and online.

Earth Friendly Products (www.ecos.com)—This environmentally minded company makes fruit and vegetable wash, ultra-concentrated liquid laundry detergent, stain and odor remover, and liquid dishwashing cleaner. The scents they use are delicious, including almond and fresh green apple. My favorite products in this line are the Parsley and the Orange Plus all purpose cleaners.

Mountain Green (www.mtgreen.com)—This popular line of cleaning products includes dishwashing liquid, laundry detergent, fabric softener, all purpose cleaner/degreaser, and glass cleaner.

Seventh Generation (www.seventhgeneration.com)—Seventh Generation's household cleaning products include a degreaser, non-chlorine bleach, glass cleaner, and carpet cleaner. Their dish soap gets rave reviews, the laundry soap doesn't add chemicals to the surface of your clothes like mainstream products, and their chlorine bleach alternative is nontoxic hydrogen peroxide. They also make non-bleached paper products, such as towels, napkins, paper plates, and bathroom tissue. These natural cleaning and paper products are sold in natural foods markets, grocery stores, co-ops, and online. Use the "store find" selection and punch in your zip code.

Tree of Life (www.goturtle.com)—Tree of Life products include automatic dishwasher concentrate, household cleaners, and other cleaning products that are widely available in natural foods stores.

For more information about creating a healthy kitchen, safe drinking water, food storage and recycling, reading food labels, and finding out how chemicals get into our food supply, review my book, *The Staying Healthy Shopper's Guide.*

APPLIANCE ADDICTION
by Bethany Argisle

There are power strips and push buttons of all kinds; we can now sit in one place and turn things on and off—but not the sun yet! Yet, we try it with one another. I have been in meetings during which everyone's cells or pagers go off, any time of day and night.

I might add that I was a child from the last pre-TV generations where there were few cars and planes and fewer expensive, symptom-of-the-month club memberships and fancy designer diseases. Our lives were much simpler, much more present. Oh sure, there were headlines and time was different, it took longer and had a sense of mystery. Now time is full before it even begins—there are alarms, there are forms online and lines everywhere—I find it amazing that with MORE, MORE, MORE, I see the word *blessing* has the word less in it.

Sure I love my electric drums, my computers, my washer and dryer, and I miss having a dishwasher that really gets my dishes clean and sparkly. In the meantime, however, I am being billed for these appliance thrills. To achieve appliancedom, then to maintain those appliances and have a stack of directions and repair numbers close by, all keeps me busy.

These appliances are a relationship, only we seem to think they give us more time for personal relationships. A recent storm in my area that hit the headlines, had me without power for a week. The sun was all I plugged into and the night told me it was time to rest. What I found very healing about this power outage was the deep silence. It seems without all those appliances on in all the houses and businesses in every direction, that a deep peace, a silence, a return to the natural became evident, until on the fifth day the neighbors all bought or rented generators—and the silence was stolen and but a brief memory of all the diseases that might stem from the violations sound produces. I notice on TV that the sounds of war particularly seem shattering to the bones of my soul.

During the power outage, another challenge became bathing. I imagined myself having to boil water for everything, but first to have to hunt and track and discover water and make it come to the surface.

Now I keep a cooking stove and candles and a hand can opener and firewood as I used to be a girl scout—let the sun light our way and rest with the darkness. Let's breathe and reconnect with Nature.

CHAPTER THIRTEEN

The Detox Diet Recipes

◆

We have expanded the options from the original version of *The Detox Diet*. We want to give you more tasty choices for foods you can consume. The following recipes are examples of foods you can eat coming off your detox program as well as some you can even consume while on your detox. We have organized them into breakfast, lunch, dinner, snacks, and drinks for easier access and application to your diet.

Part of the detoxification process is following an alkaline diet to help balance the acidic body state, which we believe leads to the toxicity and inflammation that results in the chronic, degenerative problems many westerners experience. (See earlier discussion on acid-alkaline in Chapter 2.) Therefore, our program focuses on the alkaline-generating fruits and vegetables and the most alkaline grains, which include millet, quinoa, and buckwheat. We have avoided the use of commonly reactive foods, such as wheat and dairy products other than an occasional optional ingredient, as the cheese in the Stuffed Bell Peppers (page 200).

We also suggest minimizing all chemical exposure, both from your environment and from your foods. Therefore, we support your inclusion of organic food choices whenever these are available. A review of chemical concerns and the most important foods to buy organically grown can be found in my book, *The Staying Healthy Shopper's Guide*.

Good appetite. Good food. Good health.

COOKING VEGETABLES

Before you go into the specific recipes, here are some general guidelines for cooking vegetables since they are so important to the whole process of detoxification. Focusing our diet around vegetables is a long-range health activity. The fresher the vegetables the better, with organic the best choice in order to avoid toxic chemical sprays. Cooking vegetables can make these nutritious foods easier to digest for many, but cooking can also destroy many of the health-generating vitamins and minerals from vegetables. It's important to not overcook vegetables. When steaming, allow the veggies to still have a little crunch. Furthermore, the liquid under the steamed veggies may be quite nutritious and help to alkalinize our body to rebalance us and help fight many chronic problems.

Next you will find healthy ways to prepare vegetables besides eating them raw and fresh. The methods are steaming, roasting, and water sauté. Eat a variety of four to six veggies per dish, using one or two roots only, a few less-starchy vegetables like zucchini and green beans, and some leafy greens.

Steaming

For detoxifying purposes, this is the best way to prepare vegetables. After steaming, vegetables are easy to digest and still nutritious. Simply chop your veggies into appropriate sizes for eating. Use a vegetable steamer in a large pot with a few inches of water below, or invest in a double pot with the water below and the veggies above. Start the steaming with the vegetables that take the longest time to cook; these are the hard squashes, potatoes, and roots such as carrots and beets. After 5 to 10 minutes, add the next set of veggies, such as green beans, broccoli, onions, zucchini, and the stems of chard. Finally, just before you turn off the heat, add any leafy greens to the top. Serve with the Better Butter (page 211), a splash of olive oil, and the seasonings of your choice, such as sea salt, garlic salt, cayenne pepper, or other herbs.

Roasting

To roast vegetables, preheat the oven to 325 to 350°F. Cut up the vegetables into edible strips. Slice zucchini and carrots lengthwise into quarters, cut potatoes into bite-sized pieces, and cut onions into quarters. Place all in a large bowl and pour 1 to 2 tablespoons of olive oil and mix with hands. Sprinkle on a little vegetable salt. Place in a baking pan or dish and put in the oven. After 20 minutes or so when they are browning, take out and flip the vegetables over, and cook another 10 minutes, until they are golden brown. You can also broil for a couple of minutes to add to the browning; just watch that they don't burn. Add other seasonings, if desired before serving.

Water Sauté

Begin with a hot skillet or wok and then add a splash of olive oil to the pan along with the first layer of vegetables. (As with steaming, start with the ones needing the most cooking time and add as you go.) As the veggies cook, add small amounts of water to keep them moist. Some vegetable stock/broth or a touch of wine can also be used for more flavoring. At the end, add the leafy greens, turn off the heat, and cover for a few minutes.

Note: As with all the vegetable combinations, use the best of the seasonally available choices. These usually have the best prices and since they are local, often have less treatment with chemicals. If you buy organic, there is less concern here. Shopping at local farmers' markets when available is a great option.

Seasonally Available Vegetables

~ Spring ~

Artichokes, asparagus, beets and beet greens, Brussels sprouts, chard, garlic, green onions, leeks, spinach, and wild greens.

~ Summer ~

Beets and beet greens, corn, eggplant, new potatoes, peppers, soft squashes like yellow and zucchini, and sugar snap peas.

~ Autumn ~

Bell peppers, broccoli, cauliflower, celery, corn, hard squashes (acorn, butternut, spaghetti, and so on), Jerusalem artichokes, okra, potatoes, spinach, and zucchini.

~ Winter ~

Bok choy, broccoli, cabbage, cauliflower, chard, Jerusalem artichokes, kale, hard squashes, onions, potatoes, and sweet potatoes or yams.

ADDING PROTEIN TO VEGETABLES

When you get down to a healthier long-term diet, adding some protein, such as fish or poultry to vegetable dishes is a healthy way to eat for energy, weight, and good health. For vegetarians, this can be beans and some nuts or seeds eaten along with the vegetables.

Begin with the appropriate amount of food you need for the number of people you wish to serve. Following a good diet means having foods available for you on a consistent basis. Therefore, even if you primarily eat alone, when you prepare nice dishes like these, make enough for two, three, or even four meals. You could use salmon, snapper, sea bass, or halibut, or buy a few turkey or chicken breasts. Also choose your favorite vegetables (hopefully you have many), primarily seasonally available ones as well as a mixture of low-starch ones as described previously. Some good ones to prepare with your proteins are onions, potatoes, carrots, zucchini, and mushrooms. A little white wine can be used as well as seasonings like olive oil, sea salt, soy sauce, garlic, and lemon.

Sauté or Pan Cooking

You can premarinate the strips of poultry or fish in some olive oil, tamari or sea salt, lemon, and choice of other seasonings. To a large iron skillet or wok over a medium to high heat, sauté the fish or poultry on both sides for a few minutes, and then add the vegetables as you go, the firmer ones to start. Cover the skillet for 5 to 10 minutes to allow the dish to cook throughout and merge its flavors. You may need to add a bit of water as you go to keep it moist.

There are many flavoring options for these dishes. Here are some general guidelines for flavoring.

For Asian tastes, try soy sauce, ginger, and cayenne or chili.

For Mexican flavors, use tomato, onion, cilantro, and of course, chili or cayenne peppers.

For Mediterranean tastes, add olive oil, garlic, marjoram, rosemary, and thyme.

Bon apetite!

Baking Dish Method

Place the fish or poultry in the baking dish, adding the appropriate seasonings, such as lemon, sea salt, and olive oil for the fish, or salt and herbs for the poultry. Cover and surround with the vegetables. Add a splash of water if needed to the dish to keep the food moist. Cover and place in a preheated oven at 350°F. Bake for 30 to 45 minutes. This is a full meal, yet for a more typically complete one, you can also serve with a fresh salad or some rice.

RECIPES FOR MENU PLANNING

BREAKFAST RECIPES

Basic Steel Cut Oatmeal
Hot Breakfast Quinoa
Breakfast Millet

Baked Apples
Dr. Elson's Breakfast Rice
Dani's Muesli

LUNCH AND DINNER RECIPES

Millet Pilaf
Quick Southwest Quinoa
Quinoa Tabbouleh Salad
Toasted Oat Pilaf
Stuffed Bell Peppers
Pea Hummus

Herbed Millet with Steamed Vegetables
Vegetable Curry
Lentil Stew
Salmon with Roasted Garlic and
    Rosemary

SOUPS, SALADS, AND SIDE DISHES

Herbed Soup
Gazpacho
Kombu Squah Soup
Broccoli Soup
Caraway Cabbage Borscht
Jicama Salad
White Bean Salad

Smoked Wild Salmon Salad
Asian Cucumber Salad
Glazed Broccoli
Basic or Toasted Millet
Basic Quinoa
Caramelized Onion Quinoa

SAUCES, DIPS, AND DRESSINGS

Better Butter
Tomato Vinaigrette
Parsley-Mint Sauce
Creamy Garlic Sauce
Date and Orange Chutney
Ginger Garlic Dressing

Lemon and Olive Oil Dressing
Avocado Dressing
Quick Spicy Tomato Sauce
Mango Salsa
Dr. Elson's Savory Sauce

SNACKS AND TREATS
Cold Almonds
Frozen Grapes
Mochi with Sauce
Fruit Salad with Dani's Mochi

Juice Jells
Guacamole and Vegetables
Kombu Knots
Pears in Black Cherry Sauce

HOT AND COLD DRINKS
Gingered Green Tea
Cinnamon Cider
Citrus Sparkle
Cucumber and Lemon Water
Hibiscus Tea Cooler

Apple Lemon Spritzer
Herbal teas, like Peppermint, Chamomile,
    or Lemon Grass
Coffee substitutes, like Postum, Cafix,
    or Teechino

SMOOTHIES
Ginger Cooler
Peachy Keane
Strawberry-Orange Shake
Purple Papaya
Banana Soother

Avocado Freeze
Tahini Shake
Cinnamon Pears
Strawberry Almond Shake

FRESH VEGETABLE AND FRUIT JUICES
Carrot Cocktail
After-Workout Refresher
Energizer Elixir
Cucumber Cooler
Immune Supporter

Apple Lemonade
Tropical Twist
Fresh Harvest
Sunset Soother

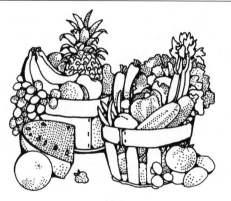

BREAKFAST RECIPES

Basic Breakfast Steel-Cut Oatmeal

Serves 3

Steel-cut oats are less processed than rolled or instant oats so they metabolize slower providing longer-lasting fuel for your body. You can add fruit to this oatmeal if you would like.

3 cups water, juice, or rice or
    oat milk
¼ teaspoon of salt

1 cup steel-cut oats
1 tablespoon maple syrup

In a saucepan, bring the water and salt to a boil over high heat. Add the steel-cut oats and return to a boil. Reduce heat to low, cover and cook 10 to 20 minutes, depending on how chewy or soft you like your cereal. Remove from the heat and let stand, covered, for a couple of minutes until slightly thickened. Serve with maple syrup.

Hot Breakfast Quinoa

Serves 4

Quinoa is delicious with toppings such as shredded coconut, raisins, and cold almonds. See the recipe on page 216 for preparing cold almonds.

1 cup quinoa
2 cups water
Salt
½ cup chopped apples, pears,
    raisins, soaked almonds, or
    dates (optional)

½ cup rice milk
1 tablespoon maple syrup
Pineapple bits, toasted shredded
    coconut, and/or ½ teaspoon
    cinnamon, for garnish (optional)

Rinse 1 cup of quinoa and drain. Place the quinoa in a saucepan over a high heat, add the water and salt, and bring to a boil. Reduce heat and simmer for 5 minutes. Add whatever fruit you desire and continue to simmer until all the water is absorbed. Serve with rice milk and a drizzle of maple syrup. Garnish with pineapple, coconut, and/or cinnamon.

Breakfast Millet

Serves 2

Millet will pick up the flavor of the sweetener. To add more protein and fiber to your breakfast, sprinkle the top with soaked almonds.

1 cup water
¼ teaspoon salt
¼ cup millet
1 cup rice milk
2 tablespoons maple syrup

Place the water, salt, and millet in a saucepan and cook over low heat for 25 to 30 minutes, until all of the water has been absorbed. Serve with rice milk; drizzle with the maple syrup.

Baked Apples

Serves 4

4 organic green apples
¼ cup raisins
8 almonds
¼ teaspoon cinnamon
2 cups water

Preheat the oven to 350°F.

Wash the apples and slice ½ an inch off the top of the apples. Set the tops aside. Core the apples with an apple corer, being careful not to puncture the bottoms of the apple. Stuff each apple with raisins, two almonds, and a sprinkle of cinnamon. Fill each apple with water and replace the tops. Transfer the apples to a baking dish and bake for 30 to 40 minutes, or until soft.

Dr. Elson's Breakfast Rice

Serves 4

1 cup raisins
1 tablespoon grated lemon zest
1 cinnamon stick or ½ teaspoon
   ground cinnamon

1 cup apple juice
4 cups cooked brown rice
½ cup coarsely chopped walnuts
   or almonds, lightly toasted

Place the raisins, lemon zest, cinnamon, and apple juice in a saucepan and simmer over low heat for 3 to 5 minutes, until the raisins are plump. Add rice and simmer a few minutes longer, turn off heat, add walnuts, and let stand, covered, for 10 minutes, or longer until all the liquid is absorbed. Serve warm.

Dani's Muesli Recipe

Serves 6

This fiber-rich breakfast cereal provides essential fatty acids and minerals that support detoxification.

2 pounds organic rolled oats
1 pound oat bran
½ pound lecithin granules
½ pound whole flaxseed
   (grind fresh)
½ pound dried raisins or currants
4 ounces raw pumpkin seeds

4 ounces pecans
6 ounces wheat germ
½ cup live culture yogurt plain
   unsweetened (optional)
1 piece of fruit, cut into small
   pieces or ½ cup berries
   (optional)

Mix all ingredients in a very large mixing bowl or a paper bag. Store in plastic bags or containers in a cool dry place. The freezer is a good place to keep a majority of the muesli. To serve, soak ½ to ¾ cup of muesli for at least a half hour in diluted fruit juice or water. If you are having digestive problems you may want to soak the muesli in water overnight to help soften the oats further.

Tips:
- Sweet crunchy apples are delicious with this recipe.
- Use a coffee grinder to grind whole flaxseed.
- To mix the ingredients, use the biggest mixing bowl you have, a large paper bag, or split the ingredients into two batches.
- Store unused muesli in your freezer in resealable plastic bags.

LUNCH AND DINNER RECIPES

Millet Pilaf

Serves 4

This flavorful dish can be modified to include your favorite vegetables. Additional vegetables can be added for color and flavor such as zucchini, carrots, or celery. Red peppers and celery are crisp, colorful additions.

1 cup millet
4 cups vegetable broth or water
1 cup chopped parsley

1 tomato, chopped
½ cup chopped green onion
Salt and black pepper

In a saucepan over low heat, combine the millet and vegetable broth, and cook for 25 to 35 minutes, until all the broth has been absorbed. Add parsley, tomato, and green onion. Season with salt and pepper. Serve warm or store in a covered container in the refrigerator for up to 4 days.

Quick Southwest Quinoa

Serves 4

Quinoa can be cooked ahead of time and kept in the refrigerator for up to 5 days. By having cooked quinoa on hand, you can whip up this dish in minutes when you don't feel like cooking.

2 cups cooked quinoa
1 cup fresh salsa
¼ cup chopped cilantro

½ a lemon or lime (optional)
Minced jalapeño, or fresh chopped
    tomato, for garnish (optional)

In a serving bowl, combine the cooked quinoa with the salsa and cilantro. Serve warm or cold. If desired, squeeze ½ of a lemon or lime over the top for a fresh tangy addition or garnish with some jalapeño or tomato.

Quinoa Tabbouleh Salad

Serves 4

Fresh parsley, mint, and lemon juice are the bright flavors that make this Lebanese dish so popular. The quinoa mingles beautifully with these flavors.

1 cup cooked quinoa
1 green onion, minced
1¼ cup minced parsley
½ cup minced fresh mint

1 tablespoon freshly squeezed
   lemon juice
1 tablespoon extra virgin olive oil
   or flaxseed oil
1 teaspoon ground cumin

Combine all ingredients and serve immediately or chill in a covered container for up to 4 days.

Stuffed Bell Pepper

Stuffed bell peppers are a meal in themselves or serve with a green or grain salad such as Quinoa Tabbouleh Salad (above).

4 green, red, or yellow bell peppers
2 teaspoons sesame oil
1 to 2 cloves garlic, minced or
   pressed
1 cup albacore tuna or cooked beans
2 cups cooked brown rice
2 green onions including green part,
   finely chopped

2 tablespoons chopped fresh
   cilantro, or 1 teaspoon ground
   coriander
1 to 2 tablespoons salsa
Sea salt
Freshly ground black pepper
4 tablespoons cheese (optional)

Preheat oven to 400°F.

Cut tops off peppers and set the tops aside. Scoop out seeds and ribs and discard. Combine the sesame oil, garlic, tuna or beans, brown rice, green onion, cilantro, and salsa in a bowl. Season with salt and pepper. Stuff the peppers with the mixture. Place the peppers on a baking sheet, right side up, and replace the pepper tops. Bake for 25 minutes. Remove the tops of the bell peppers and set aside. Sprinkle each pepper with 1 tablespoon cheese and bake for 5 more minutes until cheese is melted. Replace the pepper tops and serve immediately.

Pea Hummus

Serves 4

From Lynn McCarthy of Cottonwood Cooking School in Ketchum, Idaho. This brilliant green dip is fresh, filling, and perfect for entertaining. Serve with colorful vegetable slices as an appetizer or afternoon snack.

2 cups fresh or frozen peas
2 cloves garlic
Juice of ½ a lemon
2 tablespoons toasted tahini
Salt and freshly ground pepper
1 tablespoon ground cumin

1 tablespoon extra virgin olive oil
   (optional)
Baby carrots, celery sticks, or
   sweet red, orange, or yellow bell
   pepper slices, to serve

Mix all the ingredients in a blender or food processor until smooth. Serve in a bowl with baby carrots, celery sticks, or sliced bell pepper.

Herbed Millet with Steamed Vegetables

Serves 4

This simple, spicy dish is versatile and is a hearty accompaniment to wild salmon, a green salad, or steamed vegetables.

1 cup millet
2 cups vegetable broth or water
½ onion, finely chopped

3 small cloves garlic, peeled and
   minced
1 teaspoon chopped fresh sage

Combine all the ingredients in a saucepan over low heat. Cook for 30 to 40 minutes, until all the liquid has been absorbed. Serve warm.

Vegetable Curry

Serves 4 to 6

1 large butternut squash
2 tablespoons ghee
1 tablespoon curry powder
½ teaspoon ground cardamom
½ teaspoon ground cumin
½ teaspoon ground coriander
½ teaspoon powdered ginger
½ teaspoon asafetida (optional)
½ teaspoon anise seed
½ teaspoon turmeric

2 small onions, sliced
2 carrots, sliced diagonally
1 small cauliflower, cut into florets
1 cup green beans, cut into 2-inch
    strips
2 cups water
Sea salt
⅓ cup tahini
4 cups cooked basmati rice

Cut the butternut squash in half, remove the seeds, and cut into pieces, leaving the skin on. Transfer the squash to a large pot with water to almost cover, and boil until the pieces can be pierced with a fork. Transfer the squash to a blender or food processor and blend until puréed. Set aside.

In a heavy-bottomed saucepan, add the ghee, spices, and onion. Sauté over medium-low heat, stirring frequently, until onion is limp and spices are fragrant. Add the carrots, sauté a few minutes, add the cauliflower, sauté a few minutes longer, and then add beans. Add the water and season with salt; cover, and simmer 15 minutes. Add the tahini and puréed squash, cook, stirring, until heated through. Serve over basmati rice.

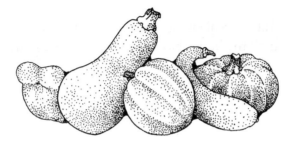

Lentil Stew

Serves 4

The addition of the seaweed kombu will aid in the digestion of the lentils.

1 cup raw lentils	1 (14 ounce) can Italian tomatoes
2 large carrots, thinly sliced	¼ teaspoon cumin powder
2 stalks celery, chopped	1 teaspoon coriander seeds
1 large onion, chopped	½ teaspoon salt
3 to 5 cloves garlic, crushed	¼ teaspoon black pepper
1 tablespoon olive oil	3 tablespoons balsamic vinegar

In a saucepan over medium heat, combine all the ingredients and cook for 30 minutes, until all the ingredients are soft.

Salmon with Roasted Garlic and Rosemary

Serves 4

This is also great cooked on the grill.

2 bulbs garlic, unpeeled
3 tablespoons freshly squeezed lemon juice
4 sprigs rosemary or 1 teaspoon dried rosemary
¼ cup extra virgin olive oil
2 (8 to 10 ounce) wild salmon fillets

Preheat oven to 350°F. Wrap the garlic bulbs loosely in aluminum foil and lay directly on oven rack. Roast the garlic for 45 minutes or until the cloves are very tender when tested with a knife. Remove the garlic from the oven and let cool. Peel the garlic, discarding the outer skin. In a food processor, combine the garlic, lemon juice, rosemary, and oil. Purée until smooth. Spread purée on the salmon. Lightly oil a baking dish with extra virgin olive oil. Transfer the salmon to a baking dish and bake until flaky, about 20 to 30 minutes.

Soups, Salads, and Side Dishes

Herbed Soup

Serves 8

10 cloves garlic, peeled and
   minced
½ cup chopped Italian parsley or
   cilantro
2 bay leaves
1 teaspoon dried sage
5 whole cloves
Pinch of dried thyme
2 quarts vegetable broth

¼ teaspoon freshly ground black
   pepper
1 (14 ounce) can stewed tomatoes
1 (16 ounce) can cooked white
   beans
Sea salt
Pinch of saffron threads
Freshly squeezed lime or lemon
   juice, to taste (optional)

Place all the ingredients except the saffron in a large stockpot and bring to a
boil. Stir well, cover, reduce heat, and simmer for 30 minutes. While the soup
is cooking, dry-roast the saffron: Heat a skillet over low heat. Add the saffron
gently, stirring constantly for 3 minutes to release the oils. Just before the soup
is finished, add the saffron to the soup, stirring to combine. Remove from the
heat, and let stand for 5 minutes. Serve warm.

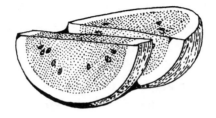

Gazpacho

Serves 8

This cold soup is not cooked and is therefore considered raw food. It is rich in antioxidants.

1 cup finely chopped red onion
2 cups seeded and finely chopped cucumber
1 cup seeded and finely diced green bell pepper
1 cup seeded and finely chopped red bell pepper
1 (28 ounce) can tomato purée
3 cloves garlic, minced
¼ cup rice wine vinegar
¼ fresh jalapeño pepper, minced
½ teaspoon freshly ground black pepper
¼ cup dry red wine or balsamic vinegar
¼ cup water
3 teaspoons freshly squeezed lime juice
3 tablespoons freshly squeezed lemon juice
1 cup finely chopped fresh cilantro

Combine all the ingredients in a large container and chill for at least 20 minutes. This cold soup can be refrigerated in an airtight container for up to 5 days. Serve chilled.

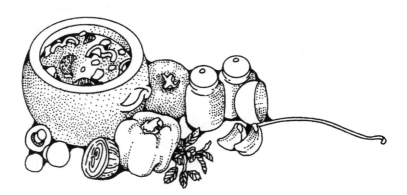

Kombu-Squash Soup

Serves 10

This is a great autumn-winter alkalizing and warming soup.

6 cups water
4 cups chopped butternut squash
1 8-inch piece kombu
1 tablespoon extra virgin olive oil
1 large onion, chopped

4 cloves garlic, minced
1 2-inch-long piece of peeled
  ginger, chopped
¼ cup balsamic vinegar
Sea salt

Bring the water to a boil in a large saucepan. Add the squash and kombu and cook over medium heat for 20 minutes. Remove the squash from the saucepan and cut away the skin. Discard the skin and return the squash to the saucepan. In a skillet, heat the olive oil over medium heat in a skillet. Add onion, garlic, and ginger and sauté for about 10 minutes. Add the sautéed vegetables to the squash mixture and cook for 1 hour, until the squash is tender. Add the balsamic vinegar, season with salt, and serve.

Broccoli Soup

Serves 4

1 (14 ounce) can vegetable or
  chicken broth
2 cups water
1 pound broccoli, chopped
1 cup sliced carrots

1 onion, sliced into rings
1 teaspoon salt
½ to 1 teaspoon coarsely ground
  black pepper (optional)

Combine the broth and water in a saucepan over high heat. Bring to a boil and add the broccoli, carrots, and onion. Season with salt and pepper. Simmer for about 30 minutes or until the vegetables are tender. For a creamier soup, blend briefly in a blender or food processor.

Caraway Cabbage Borscht

Serves 4 to 6

2 tablespoons extra virgin olive oil
2 large yellow onions, chopped
1 carrot, sliced
1 stalk celery, chopped
4 cups shredded cabbage
4 beets, cut into match sticks
2 tablespoons caraway seeds
2 teaspoons salt

Freshly ground black pepper
  (optional)
4 cups water
1 (6 ounce) can of tomato paste
2 tablespoons apple cider vinegar
1 tablespoon maple syrup
1 teaspoon dill (optional)

In a large soup pot, heat the olive oil over medium heat. Add the onion and stir over medium-high heat until caramelized. Add the carrot, celery, cabbage, beets, caraway seeds, salt, and pepper and stir well. Add the water and tomato paste and continue to cook over medium heat for 20 minutes longer. Add vinegar, maple syrup, and additional spices if desired. Serve warm or cold, or store in a glass container in the refrigerator for up to 4 days.

Jicama Salad

Serves 4

1 jicama, grated
1 carrot, grated
½ cup fresh basil leaves
⅛ to ¼ of a jalapeño pepper, grated

¼ cup chopped mint leaves
1 tablespoon freshly squeezed lime
  juice

Toss all ingredients together in a large bowl. Serve immediately.

White Bean Salad

Serves 4

1 (12 ounce) can white beans, drained	½ red onion, minced
	½ a lemon
1 cup chopped fresh Italian parsley	2 tablespoons balsamic vinegar
2 tomatoes, chopped	¼ teaspoon sea salt

In a large bowl, mix all the ingredients and serve or store, covered in the refrigerator.

Smoked Wild Salmon Salad

Serves 2

Wild salmon is a rich source of healthy oils such as Omega 3 fatty acids. Crumble over salads or cooked grains. Eat alone or dress with a drizzle of Ginger Garlic dressing.

4 cups raw salad greens
2 cups cooked quinoa, rice, or millet
½ pound smoked salmon
Ginger Garlic Dressing (page 213) or Creamy Garlic Sauce (page 212)

Place the greens in a bowl, add cooked grains if desired, crumble the salmon over, and top with a few tablespoons of dressing.

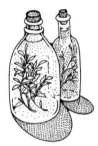

Asian Cucumber Salad

Serves 1

Tobin Jutte developed this recipe while participating in one of Daniella's detox workshops. After drinking his Indian Springs Cucumber Lemon Water, he found that the crisp cucumber slices could be made into a salad.

1 cucumber, peeled and sliced
1 tablespoon chopped red bell
  pepper
¼ cup rice wine vinegar

¼ cup water
1 tablespoon pure maple syrup
Pinch of five-spice powder and
  cayenne pepper (optional)

Combine all ingredients in a bowl, let stand for 15 minutes, and serve.

Glazed Broccoli

Serves 4

2 cups chopped broccoli
1 medium red onion, thinly sliced
1 tablespoon rice vinegar or
  balsamic vinegar

1 tablespoon brown mustard
1 tablespoon maple syrup

In a large skillet set over medium heat, steam the broccoli and onion in about 1 inch of water for 10 minutes, until tender. In a small bowl combine the vinegar, mustard, and maple syrup. Pour the maple glaze over the vegetables, and stir until evenly coated. Serve as a side dish or over cooked quinoa, rice, and/or with fish.

Basic Millet

This grain has a light delicate flavor that takes on the character of whatever it is cooked with.

1 cup millet, toasted or plain
2 cups water, juice, or vegetable broth
Salt

In a saucepan set over low heat, add the water and millet and cook for 25 to 35 minutes, until the liquid has been absorbed. Season with salt.

Toasted Millet

Serves 4

1 cup millet

In a skillet set over medium heat, add millet and cook, stirring, for 6 minutes, until the grains turn a light golden brown. Be careful not to overcook. Toasted millet can be stored for up to 2 days in the refrigerator before cooking, but it is better if used immediately.

Basic Quinoa

Serves 4

Quinoa is a versatile grain that can be used in place of rice with a stir-fry. Many people choose quinoa because it is higher in protein and provides longer-lasting energy than higher carbohydrate grains.

2 cups water, juice, or vegetable broth
1 cup quinoa
Salt

Place water and quinoa in a 2-quart saucepan and bring to a boil. Reduce to a simmer, cover, and cook until all the water is absorbed, 15 to 20 minutes. The grain should appear translucent and the germ ring will be visible. Quinoa can be toasted before cooking to give it a nutty flavor (you can toast almost any grain before cooking). To toast, place the grain in a hot, dry skillet, set over medium-high heat, stirring until it is golden brown. Be careful not to over-toast the grain. Some of the grains will "pop" during toasting, so be prepared for these hot flying missiles.

Caramelized Onion Quinoa

Serves 2

1 tablespoon extra virgin olive oil	⅓ cup quinoa
½ cup chopped onions	⅔ cup water

Add the oil and onion to a hot skillet and sauté for 5 minutes. Rinse the quinoa and add to the skillet. Add water and bring to a boil. Reduce to a simmer and continue to cook for 10 to 15 minutes or until all the water is absorbed. Serve warm as a side dish or with vegetables.

SAUCES, DIPS, AND DRESSINGS

Better Butter

Yields 2 cups

Better Butter is healthier than butter because it is made with half olive oil, so the combination has half the saturated fat and half the cholesterol of butter.

1 cup organic extra virgin olive oil (or canola or flax seed oil)
1 cup (2 sticks) organic butter, at room temperature

Combine the olive oil and butter in a glass bowl, whip together by hand, and store, covered, in the refrigerator for up to 2 weeks.

Tomato Vinaigrette

Makes 1 cup

Juice of ½ a lemon	¼ teaspoon dried thyme
1 tablespoon balsamic vinegar	¼ teaspoon dried marjoram
1 small clove garlic, minced	1 large tomato, peeled and seeded
½ teaspoon Dijon mustard	Sea salt

In a food processor or blender, combine all ingredients. Serve over seasonal mixed greens.

Parsley-Mint Sauce

Serves 4

1 onion, finely chopped
1 cup split peas
1 bay leaf
5 cups water

¼ cup minced fresh chives
1 tablespoon minced fresh mint
Sea salt

In a food processor or blender, combine all ingredients. Serve over your favorite vegetables.

Creamy Garlic Sauce

Serves 4 to 6

This is excellent over steamed vegetables, baked potatoes, or grains.

15 cloves garlic, peeled and left whole
⅛ teaspoon dried sage
⅛ teaspoon dried thyme
1½ cups water
2 tablespoons dry white wine
   (optional)

Juice of ½ a lemon
Sea salt, to taste
2 tablespoons minced parsley
Cayenne, to taste

In a saucepan, combine the garlic, sage, thyme, water, and wine. Simmer over a low heat for 20 to 30 minutes, until garlic is soft. Remove from heat, transfer mixture to a blender, and purée. Add the lemon juice and salt. Stir in the parsley and season with the cayenne. Reheat over a low flame before serving.

Note: Cayenne pepper often comes in various heat levels. It is a great warming and energizing spice that is not usually irritating. We vary in our ability to enjoy it so add to taste.

Date and Orange Chutney

Serves 4 to 6

1 whole orange, peeled and
chopped
1 cup pitted dates, chopped
1 teaspoon grated fresh ginger
⅓ cup water

⅓ cup rice vinegar
1 tablespoon brown rice syrup
¼ cup raisins
Crushed red pepper flakes to taste
Sea salt to taste

Combine all the ingredients in a saucepan. Partially cover and cook over
medium-low heat for 20 to 30 minutes until soft. This chutney keeps well in
the refrigerator for several weeks.

Ginger Garlic Dressing

Serves 8

½ an orange
1 2-inch-long piece of peeled, fresh
gingerroot
5 cloves garlic
2 tablespoons balsamic vinegar

2 tablespoons extra virgin olive oil
Juice of ¼ of a lemon
1 tablespoon tamari soy sauce or
½ teaspoon sea salt (optional)

Peel the orange by cutting off just the outside bright orange part of the peel,
leaving the inner white pithy part, which contains all of its beneficial bioflavanoids. Combine all ingredients in a blender and blend for 30 to 60 seconds.
If you prefer a creamier dressing, blend longer. To thin the dressing, add a
tablespoon of water and blend again until smooth. Serve over leafy greens,
steamed vegetables, grains, or fish.

Lemon and Olive Oil Dressing

Serves 4

This light dressing is the perfect finish for summer salads.

Juice of 1 lemon
4 tablespoons extra-virgin olive oil
Sea salt to taste

Whisk together the lemon juice, olive oil, and salt. Use to dress a salad. Or you can simplify the process and sprinkle each ingredient onto your salad separately, then toss the salad well.

Avocado Dressing

Serves 4

This is delicious over salad, grains, or beans.

2 medium avocados, peeled and
   pitted
Juice of 1 lemon
1 teaspoon salt or tamari

½ cup water
⅛ teaspoon cayenne pepper
1 clove garlic (more, if desired)

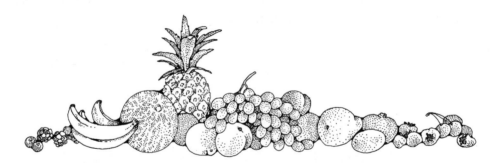

Quick Spicy Tomato Sauce

Serves 2 to 4

This rich sauce makes a hearty meal when served with fish, lentils, or cooked whole grains such as quinoa.

1 tablespoon extra virgin olive oil	1 teaspoon ground cumin
1 to 2 shallots or ½ a red onion, chopped	¼ teaspoon turmeric
2 cloves garlic, minced	½ teaspoon sea salt
1 tablespoon ground coriander	3 cups tomatoes, chopped

Heat the oil in a saucepan over medium heat. Add the shallot and garlic and sauté for 5 minutes, until soft. Add the coriander, cumin, turmeric, and salt and continue cooking, stirring, for a minute or longer, until spices are fragrant and onion begins to brown. Stir in the tomatoes, cover, and cook gently over low heat for 15 minutes, until tomatoes have turned to liquid.

Mango Salsa

Serves 6

Jalapeño peppers can vary in strength. Some are very hot and overpower the recipe. Touch the pepper with a fork and touch your tongue to the fork. This will you give you an idea of how hot your pepper is. Adjust the amount of pepper accordingly. It is also a good idea to taste the onion before adding it. The age and type of onion will alter the intensity. If you have a particularly strong onion just reduce the quantity.

1 mango, minced	1 tablespoon balsamic vinegar
½ cup chopped red bell pepper	2 tablespoons freshly squeezed lime juice
½ cup minced red onion	1 tomato, minced (optional)
1 tablespoon minced jalapeño pepper	
1 tablespoon minced fresh mint leaves	

Combine all the ingredients in a medium bowl and mix thoroughly. Serve immediately or store in a covered container in the refrigerator for up to 1 week.

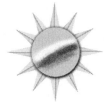

Dr. Elson's Savory Sauce

Serves 2 to 4

This can be used as a mochi dip or a sauce for grilled vegetables with rice or quinoa.

2 tablespoons almond butter or
    tahini
1 tablespoon organic miso paste
1 tablespoon honey

1 tablespoon water (or to
    preferred consistency)
1 pinch cayenne pepper or to taste

Combine and stir all ingredients with a fork, adding until you have your desired texture and cayenne to taste.

SNACKS AND TREATS

Cold Almonds

Serves 6

Soaking nuts helps to soften their fiber making them easier to digest. They taste fresh and cool and make an easy to grab snack for those on the run. This process works with all nuts such as cashews, hazelnuts, or walnuts.

1 pound organic raw almonds
Filtered water

Pour almonds into a large bowl and cover with filtered water. Soak for at least 4 hours. Keep the nuts in the water until they are eaten. Use as a snack or to top oatmeal and other cooked grains.

Frozen Grapes

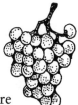

1 bunch of organic grapes

Wash grapes and remove from stem. (If seeds, eating some are healthful.) Pat the grapes dry and place then in a zip lock bag in the freezer. Frozen grapes make the perfect snack on hot days and a nice addition to fruit or green salads, or as ice cubes in drinks.

Mochi with Sauce

1 package of Mochi
Optional: Honey, better butter, nut butter, or maple syrup

Mochi is essentially compressed, cooked, brown rice. It is sold in a variety of sweet or savory flavors. Follow the directions for baking listed on the package. As the mochi bakes it rises forming a pastry that is chewy on the inside and crunchy on the outside—simple and yet so decadent. The cinnamon mochi begs for a dab of better butter and a drizzle of honey or maple syrup to serve as a dessert or with tea. The savory flavors can be served as part of a meal or as a snack and can be filled with garlic sautéed in better butter. All can be eaten with a bit of Dr. Elson's Savory Sauce (page 216).

Fruit Salad with Dani's Muesli

Serves 1

½ cup dark berries (blueberries or blackberries)
½ cup apple, banana, or other favorite fruit
¼ to ½ cup Dani's Muesli (page 198)
¼ cup organic yogurt (optional)

Wash berries and place in bowl. Add chopped melon and top with Muesli and yogurt if desired. This high fiber, antioxidant-rich treat makes a hearty snack, or a refreshing breakfast alternative.

Juice Jells

> 2 cups fresh fruit juice (apple, berry, cranberry, grape, and so on)
> 1 to 2 teaspoons of agar

Combine the juice and agar flakes in a saucepan and let stand for 2 to 3 minutes. Bring the juice to a simmer over low heat and cook, stirring, for about 10 minutes, until agar is dissolved. Continue stirring the mixture over low heat for 5 minutes longer. Transfer to serving dishes and chill in the refrigerator for at least 2 hours, until thickened. Serve cold or frozen as Popsicles.

Guacamole and Vegetables

> *Serves 4*

2 ripe medium to large avocados, minced
2 ripe small to medium tomatoes, minced
3 cloves garlic, minced or 1 teaspoon garlic powder
3 tablespoons freshly squeezed lemon or lime juice

1 teaspoon balsamic vinegar
¼ red onion, minced
4 cups sliced raw vegetables such as baby carrots, zucchini slices, and orange, red, and yellow bell peppers

In a serving bowl, mash all the ingredients together using a fork. Serve with crunchy vegetables.

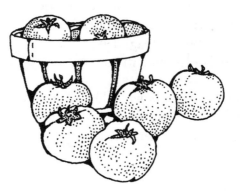

Kombu Knots

Serves 4 to 8

Kombu has a naturally salty flavor that lends just the right flavor to this potato chip-like snack. Seaweeds help alkalinize the body.

1 package of kombu seaweed
Extra virgin olive oil, for cooking

Soak the kombu in water to soften. Using scissors, cut the kombu into long strips about ⅛-inch wide and 3 inches long. Tie the strips into simple knots. Pour the oil into a small saucepan to a depth of up to 1 inch. Set over medium-high heat until the oil is hot, but not smoking. Drop the kombu knots into oil, making sure they are submerged, and cook for about 1 minute each. Transfer to a paper towel to drain.

Pears in Black Cherry Sauce

Serves 4

4 firm pears
1 2-inch piece of peeled fresh ginger, cut into matchsticks or 1
  tablespoon grated fresh ginger

4 cups black cherry juice
3 tablespoons kudzu diluted in
  4 tablespoons cold water
4 sprigs mint, for garnish

Place pears and ginger in large, heavy-bottom pot and add the cherry juice. The juice should half-cover the pears and ginger. Cover and simmer over low heat, until pears are soft but not mushy, piercing with a toothpick to test for doneness. Remove pears from the pot, reserving the juice, and transfer the pears to individual serving plates. Add dissolved kudzu to simmering juice and stir over low heat until thickened. Pour 1 cup of the sauce over each pear and garnish with a mint sprig.

HOT AND COLD DRINKS

Gingered Green Tea

Serves 1

Green tea naturally contains some caffeine. Buy decaffeinated green tea if you prefer. Ginger is a gentle remedy for upset stomach and is warming on cold mornings.

1 green tea bag
Filtered water
½-inch-long piece of fresh ginger, sliced

Place the teabag in a mug of hot water with 2 to 3 slices of ginger and serve.

Cinnamon Cider

Serves 2

This slightly more exotic version of hot apple cider has subtle flavors of India and a hint of maple.

2 cups unsweetened apple cider or apple juice
¼ teaspoon ground cinnamon
¼ teaspoon ground ginger
2 teaspoons maple syrup
½ an orange, sliced
¼ teaspoon of ground cardamom (optional)
Fresh, peeled ginger slices (optional)

In a saucepan, heat the apple cider over low heat in a saucepan. Add cinnamon, ginger, maple syrup, and any other spices desired to the cider. Place orange slices in the mug and add cardamom and fresh ginger, if you like. Pour hot cider into mugs and serve hot.

Citrus Sparkle

Serves 2

Use bottled sparkling water without additives or chemicals such as Calistoga mineral water or Perrier.

2 sweet citrus fruits such as orange or pink grapefruit
2 cups sparkling mineral water

Use a paring knife to remove the outer colored part of the fruit peel and be sure to leave the white pithy inner layer intact, as it is rich in bioflavanoids. Combine in a blender until smooth and serve immediately.

Cucumber and Lemon Water Indian Springs Health Elixir

Makes 1 gallon

This light refreshing drink is so tasty you'll be inspired to drink water all day long.

1 cucumber, peeled and cored
1 lemon, sliced
1 gallon purified water or mineral water

Cut the cucumber into 4 long strips and place in a glass pitcher with the lemon slices. Cover with water and ice if desired. The cucumber and lemon will last all day. After you finish drinking the water just add more to the pitcher.

Hibiscus Tea Cooler

Serves 2

This drink is light and only slightly sweet and can be made with a variety of juices.

1 hibiscus tea bag
1 cup hot water
1 cup cranberry juice

Steep the tea bag in the hot water until desired potency. Chill tea in the refrigerator or add ice to cool. Combine with cranberry juice or berry juice of choice.

Apple Lemon Spritzer

Serves 2

2 apples
1 lemon (or lime)
2 cups sparkling mineral water

Use a paring knife to remove the outer colored part of the lemon peel and be sure to leave the white pithy inner layer intact, as it is rich in bioflavanoids. Add the apple and lemon to your juicer and juice according to the manufacturer's instructions. Pour into glasses with mineral water and serve with lemon wedges.

Herbal Teas

Chamomile
Peppermint
Pau D' Arco
Hibiscus

Lemon grass
Ginger root
Red clover

HERBS YOU MAY FIND IN DETOX FORMULAS

Cascara sagrada
Senna leaves
Rhubard root
Licorice root
Ginger root
Burdock root
Dandelion root and leaf
Black cohosh root
Barberry root
Buckthorn bark
Cinnamon bark
Slippery elm bark
Psyllium seeds
Bentonite clay
Apple pectin
Juniper berry

Fennel seed
Milk thistle seed
Nettle leaf
Red clover flower
Peppermint leaf
Golden seal
Sheep sorrel
Watercress
Aloe vera
Artichoke leaf
Sodium alginate
Prickly ash bark
Fenugreek seed
Schizandra berry
Long pepper berry
Clove bud

GRAIN BEVERAGES FOR COFFEE SUBSTITUTES

Grain drink mixes are made of ingredients such as malt, chicory, barley, rye, figs, beet roots, and licorice. Add rice, hazelnut, or grain milks for a latte-like replacement drink.

Pioneer
Rostaroma
Cafix

Barley Coffee
Inka
Pero

Rombouts
Raja's Cup
Wilson's Heritage

SMOOTHIES

Smoothies are a creative and nourishing way to support your detoxification. Here are some tasty combinations to help you get started. You can also customize smoothies to fit your nutritional needs and taste. We have included a smoothie ingredient list just after the recipes to help you find the right combination to provide energy and nutrients while you satisfy sweet flavor in a balanced way. Smoothies can also be added to the Detox Diet for those who want to support their weight.

Ginger Cooler

Serves 1

1 apple, cored, peeled, and sliced
½ cup filtered water
½ cup ice

1 lemon, peeled, halved, and seeded
1 2-inch-long piece of peeled, fresh
   ginger, crushed

Combine all the ingredients in a blender and drink immediately.

Peachy Keane

Serves 1

1 cup orange juice
1 cup fresh peaches or drained
   canned peaches

2 tablespoons vanilla protein powder
1 teaspoon natural yeast
Greens powder, flax oil (optional)

Combine all the ingredients in a blender and drink immediately.

Strawberry-Orange Shake

Serves 1

1 cup orange juice
1 cup frozen organic strawberries
1 frozen organic banana

200 mg vitamin C powder, protein
   powder, greens powder, flax oil
   (optional)

Combine all the ingredients in a blender and drink immediately.

Purple Papaya

Serves 1

1 cup purple grape juice
1 cup fresh or frozen papaya slices
Protein powder, greens powder, flax oil (optional)

Combine all the ingredients in a blender and drink immediately.

Banana Soother

Serves 1

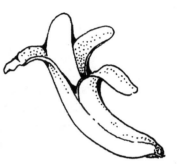

1 cup rice milk
1 frozen banana
4 mint leaves
Protein powder, greens powder, flax oil (optional)

Combine all the ingredients in a blender and drink immediately.

Avocado Freeze

Serves 1

½ avocado, peeled, pitted, and
   sliced
1 tablespoon freshly squeezed
   lemon juice
1 cup frozen cherries, pitted
1 cup orange juice
Protein powder, greens powder,
   flax oil (optional)

Combine all the ingredients in a blender and drink immediately.

Tahini Shake

Serves 2

1 cup rice milk	2 tablespoons tahini
1 cup orange juice	Protein powder, greens powder,
1 frozen banana	flax oil (optional)

Combine all the ingredients in a blender and drink immediately.

Cinnamon Pears

Serves 2

2 pears, peeled and cored or use canned pears
½ cup orange juice
1 teaspoon ground cinnamon
Protein powder, greens powder, flax oil (optional)

Combine all the ingredients in a blender and drink immediately.

Tobin's Strawberry Almond Shake

Serves 1

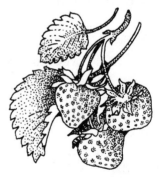

½ cup almond milk
½ cup strawberries, frozen and preferably organic
2 tablespoons maple syrup

Blend all the ingredients in a blender and serve immediately.

SMOOTHIE INGREDIENT OPTIONS

Adapted from *Smoothies for Life* by Daniella Chace and Maureen Keane (Prima Publishing, 1998)

Beneficial Microflora

Acidophilus and Bifidus are two well-known organisms that are an important part of a healthy gut flora. Hundreds of similar organisms have now been identified that function in our intestines to help us digest our food completely, absorb natural beneficial hormones from plants, and fight off bad bacteria and viruses. Primal Defense (Garden of Life product) or other microflora replacement powders can be purchased at health food stores, grocery stores, and many pharmacies.

Avocados

The avocado is one of the richest plant sources of glutathione, a potent antioxidant that can detoxify environmental pollutants. It also contains vitamin E, another antioxidant, and enough oil to ensure that this fat-soluble vitamin is absorbed.

Brewer's Yeast

Nutritional yeast or brewer's yeast can be added to smoothies in small amounts without altering the flavor drastically. Add one teaspoon of either yeast powder to a smoothie to add folic acid, pyridoxine (vitamin B_6), and vitamin B_{12}.

Chlorella

This blue-green algae is used in the detoxification of heavy metals such as cadmium, uranium, and lead. Studies in Japan have shown that chlorella increases the excretion of cadmium from victims of cadmium poisoning. Chlorella contains many nutrients, especially amino acids, which support mental and physical energy and detoxification. Powdered chlorella is available at health food stores. Start by adding just one teaspoon to your smoothies and then add more if you like the flavor.

Greens Powders

These are generally made of various algaes and chlorophyll (from barley grass or wheat grass, for example), which provide minerals, trace minerals, and antioxidants to help remove free radicals from your body. For example: Perfect Food (Garden of Life product), ProGreens (Nutricology), Barleans Greens, and Green Vibrant.

Milk Alternatives

Grain, bean, and nut milks can be used in place of dairy milk. There are many available in the stores such as oat milk, rice drink, almond milk, hazelnut milk, soy milk, multi-grain milk, and so forth. These products are sold in cartons and in aseptic boxes that do not require refrigeration. There are many varieties such as vanilla, chocolate, low-fat, and organic. Buy organic to be sure the product is free of agricultural chemicals, and avoid the ones with flavor added as they are generally higher in sugar than their plain counterparts.

Nut Butters

Peanut butter, which is ground peanuts, is just one of the many nut butters. Cashew butter, almond butter, hazelnut butter, and even pistachio butter are now available. Buy high-quality nut butters without sugar, preservatives, or hydrogenated oils. Maranatha and Kettle are two brands that are of good quality.

Protein Powders

The protein in these powders is often from soybeans, which means you should look for organic soy protein powder or if that is not available then look for non-GMO on the label. Non-GMO (Genetically Modified Organism) indicates that the product is not genetically engineered. If you tolerate dairy, whey powders are popular and widely available. Rice protein is also available and hemp seed protein has just hit the stores.

Psyllium Seed

Psyllium seeds are rich sources of soluble fiber called mucilage. The mucilage in psyllium seed aids in colon health and it prevents constipation and binds cholesterol and toxins in the intestine. When added to water, psyllium seed powder can swell to ten times its original size. It is odorless and bland in taste but has a gritty texture that is reduced by adding it to a drink containing frozen fruit. Start with one teaspoon of psyllium seed powder and gradually work up to one tablespoon, to avoid developing gas. Drink a lot of water when you consume psyllium.

Soluble Fiber

Psyllium seed powder, flaxseed powder, oat bran, and pectin are all soluble fiber sources that can be added to smoothies. Start with one teaspoon, working gradually up to one tablespoon. Soluble fiber is a type of carbohydrate that resists digestion by gastrointestinal secretions. It dissolves in the watery contents of the small intestine, producing a viscous gel. Soluble fiber binds toxins in the colon. It also will decrease the chance of constipation and lower cholesterol levels.

FRESH VEGETABLE AND FRUIT JUICES

Carrot Cocktail

Serves 1

4 carrots
Handful of spinach
Handful of parsley
½ an apple

Add all ingredients to your juicer and juice according to the manufacturer's instructions. Serve immediately.

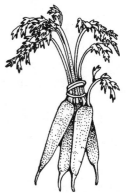

After Workout Refresher

Serves 1

4 carrots
2 stalks celery
1 apple
Handful of parsley

Add all ingredients to your juicer and juice according to the manufacturer's instructions. Serve immediately.

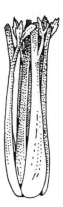

Energizing Elixir

Serves 1

2 slices of pineapple, with skin
½ cucumber
½ apple, seeded

Add all ingredients to your juicer and juice according to the manufacturer's instructions. Serve immediately.

Cucumber Cooler

Serves 1

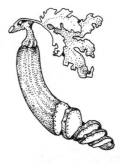

1 cucumber
1 apple
2 stalks celery
1 lemon wedge (optional)

Add all ingredients to your juicer and juice according to the manufacturer's instructions. Serve immediately.

Immune Supporter

Serves 1

3 broccoli florets
1 clove garlic
4 carrots
Handful of spinach

Add all ingredients to your juicer and juice according to the manufacturer's instructions. Serve immediately.

Apple Lemonade

Serves 1

You can add cucumber or celery to this recipe to increase the electrolytes. Any apple variety will be delicious in this juice combination but Fuji apples are exceptionally tasty.

3 apples
½ a lemon

Add all ingredients to your juicer and juice according to the manufacturer's instructions. Serve immediately.

Tropical Twist

Serves 1

Lime juice over fresh papaya slices is a wonderful treat and just as tasty in this juice.

1 papaya, peeled
¼-inch-slice of peeled, fresh ginger
1 lime wedge

Add all ingredients to your juicer and juice according to the manufacturer's instructions. Serve immediately.

Fresh Harvest

Serves 1

2 cloves garlic
Handful of greens (kale, collards, spinach, and so on)
1 tomato
2 stalks celery

Juice according to your machines' instructions and serve immediately.

Sunset Soother

Serves 1

1 cup cherries
1 bunch grapes
1 lemon wedge

Use a paring knife to remove the outer colored part of the lemon peel and be sure to leave the white pithy inner layer intact. Add all ingredients to your juicer and juice according to the manufacturer's instructions. Serve immediately.

RECIPE REFERENCES

Many of the recipes we have included in this book are favorites of ours from previous books. We have listed those titles for those of you who would like to learn more about cooking with whole foods.

From *The What to Eat if You Have Diabetes Cookbook*, by Daniella Chace and Maureen Keane

Kombu-Squash Soup
Lentil Stew
Jicama Salad
Mango Salsa
Herbed Soup
White Bean Salad
Gazpacho

Recipe adapted from *The What to Eat if You Have Cancer Cookbook* by Maureen Keane and Daniella Chace

Glazed Broccoli
Salmon with Roasted Garlic and Rosemary

Adapted from *The RV Cookbook* by Amy Boyer and Daniella Chace

Guacamole

Recipes adapted from *Grains for Better Health* by Maureen Keane and Daniella Chace

Quick Southwest Quinoa
Quinoa Tabbouleh Salad
Hot Breakfast Quinoa
Caramelized Onion Quinoa
Quinoa Tabbouleh Salad

Recipes adapted from *Smoothies for Life* by Daniella Chace and Maureen Keane

Cinnamon Pears
Tahini Shake
Banana Soother
Avocado Freeze
Purple Papaya
Strawberry-Orange Shake
Peachy Keane

Recipes adapted from *A Cookbook for All Seasons*, by Dr. Elson Haas

Caraway Cabbage Borscht
Quick Spicy Tomato Sauce
Creamy Garlic Sauce
Parsley-Mint Sauce
Tomato Vinaigrette
Pears in Black Cherry Juice

Recipes adapted from *The False Fat Diet* by Elson Haas

Breakfast Rice
Avocado Dressing
Broccoli Soup

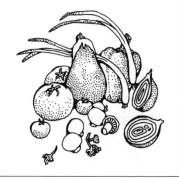

Special Needs and Healing Seeds

SPECIAL NEEDS

Menstrual Periods

During their menses, women tend to feel colder, more depleted, and weaker as they are losing blood and iron. It's a time (or should be) of pulling in and caring for oneself. However, it is also a cleansing time of the month and some women feel better during and after their periods when they do not eat too much or too heavily and are doing a mild detox program. Although we do not recommend fasting, drinking additional nutrient-rich juices can be helpful. For women who are generally in good health, the Detox Diet and the Smoothie Cleanse can be helpful. We suggest adding some algae and protein powders during this time for more energy and strength.

Menopause

During the menopause transition, there are many shifts and changes, problems with moods and sleep, and variations in body temperatures. With all of these changes going on, a detoxification program can be quite helpful as long as the woman is not weak and depleted. Doing a week or two of one of the programs in this book may help improve energy, moods, sleep, and make the menopause transition easier. You can also tell what symptoms come from congestion and toxicity and what may be hormone changes. When we finish a detox period, our body often works much better.

Pregnancy and Nursing

We generally do not recommend any intense detox programs during pregnancy and the first six months of breastfeeding when the mother is typically the sole source of her child's nutrition. A balanced diet full of good quality and nutrient-rich foods is the usual plan, and this is best made up of the wholesome foods that comprise the non-toxic diet discussed in this book—lots of fresh fruit and vegetables, whole grains and beans, nuts and seeds, fish and other good protein foods, while avoiding the junk foods. Enhancing the diet with fresh juices and smoothies is no problem and provides the additional nourishment needed during pregnancy and nursing. You can see more on these topics in Chapter 15 of my book, *Staying Healthy with Nutrition*.

Elderly

The state of nourishment, energy, weight, and health issues of the elder will determine the appropriate diet and detoxification program. We have many people in their sixties and seventies in our groups and they can do very well. There is not usually any age issues when it comes to cleaning up the body and creating a more healthful nourishment plan. It helps all of us. However, as with any age, if the person is underweight, fatigued, or malnourished in any way, it is wise that the diet be more complete and nourishing. That said, doing the Detox Diet with some added protein for a week or two can be a useful transition to a healthier and more well-rounded way of eating. Adding a smoothie once or twice a day is another way to add more nourishment and build up the body's weight and strength.

Children

Ideally, children start their lives with clean and healthy food. It saddens me to see a five or ten year old walking around with a can of Pepsi or Coke, not realizing that the hooks of caffeine and sugar will become so strong and potentially addictive. Furthermore, these unhealthy foods provide no nourishment and over-stimulation that leads often to energy and mood disorders. ADHD (Attention-Deficit Hyperactivity Disorder) has become common and is definitely connected to children's diet choices. It's wise to do something about this early as parents act more preventively to help their children make better choices. And this starts by setting a good example.

Even though we believe in freedom of choice for what we each do to our own bodies, it is up to the parents and the government to set nutritional guidelines and not let large corporations overrun and pressure legislature in regard to our food availability. We need to have the junk foods, chips, sodas, candies, and other sweets reflect the cost to the society's health and health care system as it now does with alcohol and nicotine. This is currently called "the snack tax," or maybe a better term is "the treat tax" and we need to limit our treats for best health. Educating and empowering young people toward lifelong good health begins by learning and being supported in positive lifestyle actions. Let's make that a high priority in family life.

Children, like most people, need a balanced and nourishing diet. Cleaning up the bad habits, getting off sugar and caffeine, and in some cases (like for recurrent ear infections) getting off milk products and wheat (to see if health improves) are all healthful nutritional approaches in pediatric care. Adapting the guidelines in this book provides a useful tool to our youngsters in getting them on a healthier plan for life. Remember, it can be fun to be healthy. Be positive with young ones. Offer alternatives to unhealthy foods and don't criticize. And please take an active role in school lunches and what kids do with their friends or at parties. As difficult as it sounds, discovering healthful living can be a joyous experience.

Fatigue, Anemia, and Hypothyroidism

These issues are often correlated with depletion, coldness of the body, lack of endurance, and fatigue. When people who have these conditions fast or consume a deficient diet for very long, they may get worse. They certainly can follow a detox plan away from the SNACCs or off of refined flour and other wheat and sugar products, even avoiding dairy, corn, soy, or other foods that could be causing reactions. The key here is to include other nourishing and caloric foods like nuts and seeds, grains and legumes, and fresh vegetables. Some animal proteins may be helpful as well.

Weight Loss

Even though detoxifying our body and cleaning up our health-undermining habits is useful for everyone, when we limit our diet and follow the programs outlined in this book, we may lose weight. If you are already normal or underweight, this is not ideal. Therefore, we have addressed this issue in the text. In summary, you can create a detox program that adds additional calories and meals. This can include additional smoothies and fresh vegetable juices in between meals, as well as some nuts and seeds, and grains and/or beans added to the vegetable meals. If the calorie count stays similar to your usual diet, your weight should be maintained.

Diabetes and Low Blood Sugar

Blood sugar issues can be well handled during detox and cleansing programs if people consume calories at least every two to three hours during the day. It's best not to do fasting with juices that are high in sugars, such as apple, orange, and carrots. With a high fruit and vegetable diet, it's good to add some amino acids, protein powder, or blue-green algae, which is high in nutrients and amino acids. I have had many patients with diabetes and low blood sugar do fine with detox programs since the calorie intake is lower than usual and the food choices are typically healthier. Other supplements can be used to balance the sugar issues, such as the blue-green algae just mentioned, as well as protein powders, the minerals chromium and vanadium, adrenal glandular, B vitamins, and vitamin C. Juice cleansing with diabetes needs to be done with caution (especially with insulin dependence) and with an experienced medical guide.

Heart and Blood Vessel Disease

I believe that the detoxification process can prevent, or at least delay, the incidence and progression of blood vessel atherosclerosis and subsequent heart disease. Inflammation and acidity are deeper primary factors in creating arterial plaque. We can minimize this process and improve our chances to avoid the plaque and the decreased circulation, high blood pressure, and heart attacks and strokes that can follow. Our overall more alkaline diet, high in vegetable foods, will keep the cholesterol down as well as the blood viscosity (thickness). With a lower incidence of atherosclerosis, high blood pressure, and high cholesterol, along with a high fiber, nutrient-rich diet and regular exercise, and we have the basis for a long and healthy, and vital, life.

Cancer

The above heart disease prevention plan may also help prevent cancer. The only sensible approach to cancer is prevention, as there is no generally great or effective treatment. Lifestyle (for our body and our planet) is the key to this prevention, and this begins with not smoking and avoiding most environmental and food chemicals. Nutritional balance with wholesome food and avoiding physical and persistent emotional stress helps. Likewise, the process of detoxification as described in this book works much better in cancer prevention I believe than it does in treatment. When someone is ill with cancer, whether it's right to fast and detoxify or nourish oneself in a balanced way, should be a special part of a whole program overseen by someone experienced in treating cancer.

Mercury Toxicity

Mercury is a toxic metal that is so common these days and a great concern for the nervous system, that's the brain and all the nerves. We are all exposed nowadays to mercury from ocean fish, dental amalgam fillings (still!), and other areas of environment. The detoxification of mercury and other heavy metals, such as lead, cadmium, and arsenic, is a full and separate discussion. There are several books and some new ones coming from my dentist friend and associate, Dr. Tom McGuire. The more general detoxification programs within this book will support mercury and other toxin elimination, which also happens whenever we avoid the intake of these substances, as our body is always detoxifying metals and chemicals it has stored and doesn't like. Thus, a good part of mercury detox is in avoiding it and supporting the body's elimination process. Natural products like cilantro and alginates (from seaweeds) are helpful, and medical prescriptions include DMSA and DMPS. Consult with your naturally oriented practitioner about mercury evaluation and detoxification.

Emotional Issues/Challenges

Detoxification (and toxicity) occurs at every level of our being. When we go through detox programs as outlined in this book, we may feel differently, both within us and in our relationships at work, home, and with our loved ones. We want you to be aware that this is part of the challenge of the healthy detoxification process. What can you do besides eating what you have been used to, or when you are not smoking or consuming caffeine and sugar? And what if others in your home have not changed and you feel restricted and weakened by their habits? The greatest goal of detoxification programs is to not revert to old destructive habits, instead creating new ways of healthier living. Keep aligned with your new goals and ask for support from others in your environment.

Detox and Travel

Ideally it's best to be home when we are doing any detox programs to lower the stress and to make life easier. We can then better follow our program with the right foods and supplements. Saying that, it is also possible to be away from home and still follow some basic guidelines, like being off of sugar and caffeine, even off of dairy and wheat, although it's more difficult when we're on the move or in places without that awareness. Most packaged and fast foods have all the basic junk—refined flour and sugar, as well as other toxic components. Buying whole foods and eating at healthier restaurants allows us to follow this better.

Detox and Restaurants

Although restaurant eating is often a challenge when it comes to avoiding sugar, salt, fats, wheat, cow's milk, and so on, it still can be done. Asking for what you want and letting the waitperson know you have "allergies" to certain items will often help. You can always get a good salad, rice and veggies, fish or poultry and vegetables. You might suggest that your dressings and sauces be served on the side and try the dish with your taste buds first before you enhance or cover up the natural flavors. Even lettuce can be spicy or bitter, and broccoli can taste green and nourishing when lightly steamed. I have a full review of what to look for and ideas for selections at a wide variety of restaurants in my book, *The Staying Healthy Shopper's Guide,* and on my website, www.elsonhaas.com.

Miso and Yogurt

These are the best of soy and dairy. Part of detoxification and maintaining good health means taking a break from commonly used foods, like wheat and sugars, cow's milk, and soy foods. Many people react adversely from these foods for a wide variety of reasons. This book does not include the common toxins of usually reactive foods. However, if you are going to enjoy any dairy products, we recommend the naturally fermented one, such as organic low-fat or nonfat yogurt, or miso, which is a fermented soybean paste used to make soups, dressings, and sauces. There are many types of misos, from white to dark, and from a light to strong taste. Tempeh, another fermented whole soy food, is a nourishing vegetarian protein.

Liver Detox

Our liver is always detoxifying various chemicals we are exposed to as well as the substances we create that need to be eliminated or transformed. It also produces thousands of substances our body uses. Thus, it has a lot of responsibility and doesn't really appreciate us being less responsible with our food and substance choices that make the liver's work more difficult. Alcohol and petroleum byproducts are common concerns. We support their removal with general detoxification programs as outlined in this book to provide the liver with plenty of detox support. There are many products in the natural food stores that focus, or say they focus, on the liver. Herbs such as dandelion root and leaf, burdock root, and milk thistle are safe and helpful.

Gall Bladder Flushes

There is a commonly suggested and misunderstood naturopathic practice that purports to dump many hundreds to thousands of gallstones from the gall bladder. It prescribes a combination of lemon juice and olive oil taken in the morning along with lying on one's side and massaging the belly. Then it suggests that we pass many white stone-like pebbles in our stool. And wow, look at all those gallstones! The problem is, these are not stones at all, but coagulated pieces of oil and cholesterol and whatever else forms these dissolvable and crushable "stones." The gall bladder and liver flushes may offer some remedy, however, not in clearing stones.

HEALING SEEDS

What are Healing Seeds, or what is healing for that matter? Since we used that title above, I will suggest these above items are positive thoughts that inspire improved lifestyle choice and then, improved health. Disease and healing occur at all levels of our being and are totally affected by how we live our lives as well as our genetics and early upbringing. It's difficult to make changes in habits without addressing emotional reasons and challenges to become more aware and whole. I wish you good changes and great results. Please explore deeper philosophies and approaches in my book, *Staying Healthy with the Seasons*, and on my website, www.elsonhaas.com.

Resource Roundup

◆

We have added this Resource Roundup for those of you who may have certain conditions and concerns, as well as for those who have a difficult time detoxing. We have listed reference books, hotlines, and other pertinent information.

We have also listed several options for ordering special foods. If you do not have access to healthful detox products, you may order them online. If and when you wish to go on a detox retreat—at a spa or with a qualified medical practitioner, you may do further research from our basic categories. A yoga and detoxifying diet retreat is a good balance for restoring your body and life, as is taking a break from electromagnetic vibes and the phone zone, your habits and temptations, or just bopping and shopping around town.

NOTE: See the Resource Guide in the new edition of *Staying Healthy with the Seasons* for more guidance on finding practitioners and health facilities.

When you discover other info, please e-mail it through www.elsonhaas.com.

BIBLIOGRAPHY

Baker, Sidney MacDonald, M.D. and Jean Barilla (Editor). *Detoxification & Healing*. New York: NTC Contemporary Book/McGraw Hill, 1998.

Bennett, Peter, N.D. and Barrie Stephen, N.D. *7-Day Detox Miracle*. Roseville, CA: Prima Publishing, 2001.

Bland, Dr. Jeffrey. *The 20-Day Rejuvenation Diet Program*. New Canaan, CT: Keats Publishing, Inc., 1996.

Blumenthal, Mark et al. *The ABC Clinical Guide to Herbs*. Austin, TX: American Botanical Council, 2003.

Casdorph, H. Richard, M.D., and Morton Walker, M.D. *Toxic Metal Syndrome: How Metal Poisonings Can Affect Your Brain*. Garden City Park, NY: Avery Publishing Group, 1995.

Chace, Daniella and Maureen Keane. *Smoothies for Life*. Roseville, CA.: Prima Publishing, 1998.

Cousens, Gabriel, M.D. *Spiritual Nutritional and the Rainbow Diet*. San Rafael, CA: Cassandra Press, 1986.

Dadd, Debra Lynn. *Nontoxic Home and Office: Protecting Yourself and Your Family from Every-day Toxins and Health Hazards,* revised edition. Los Angeles: Jeremy P. Tarcher, 1992.

Dadd, Debra Lynn. *Nontoxic, Natural, and Earthwise: How to Protect Yourself from Harmful Products and Live in Harmony with the Earth*. Los Angeles: Jeremy P. Tarcher, 1990.

Dufty, William. *Sugar Blues*. New York: Warners, 1966.

Furman, Joel, M.D. *Fasting and Eating for Health*. New York: St. Martin's Press, 1995.

Gittleman, Ann Louise. *Guess What Came to Dinner: Parasites and Your Health*. Garden City Park, NY: Avery Publishing Group, 1993.

Krohn, Jaclyn. *Natural Detoxification,* Updated and Expanded Edition. Francis Taylor Hartley & Marks Publishers, 2001.

Rapp, Doris, M.D. *Chemical Time Bomb*. Buffalo, NY: Environmental Research Foundation, 2003.

Reno, Liz and Joanna Devrais. *Allergy-Free Eating*. Berkeley, CA: Celestial Arts, 1995.

Shelton, Herbert. *Fasting Can Save Your Life*. Tampa, FL: American Natural Hygiene Society, 1978.

Silver, Helene. *Body Smart System: The Complete Guide to Cleansing and Rejuvenation,* Revised Edition. Sonora, CA: Healthy Healing, 1995.

Szekely, Edmund Bordeaux. *The Essene Gospel of Peace. Book 1*. San Diego, CA: Academy Books, 1977.

Tompkins, Peter, and Christopher Bird. *Secrets of the Soil*. New York: Harper Collins, 1989.

The following books are currently out of print, and they were used in the writing of the original *Detox Diet*. They may still be helpful and insightful in your health pursuit. You might find them on Amazon or in a used bookstore.

Aero, Rita and Stephanie Rick. *Vitamin Power: A User's Guide to Nutritional Supplements and Botanical Substances That Can Change Your Life*. New York: Harmony Books, 1987.

Airola, Paavo. *How to Get Well*. Phoenix, AZ: Health Plus, 1981.

Ferguson, Tom, M.D. *Smoker's Book of Health: How to Keep Yourself Healthier and Reduce Your Smoking Risks*. New York: G. P. Putnam's Sons, 1987.

Saifer, Phyllis, M.D. *Detox*. Los Angeles, CA: Jeremy P. Tarcher, 1984.

Yogananda, Paramahansa. *Healing by God's Unlimited Power*. Los Angeles, CA: Self Realization Fellowship, 1975.

LABORATORIES FOR DETOXIFICATION AND GASTROINTESTINAL TESTING

ACCU-CHEM Laboratories
990 N. Bowser Rd., Suite #880
Richardson, TX 75081
800-747-2878

This lab measures chemical toxicity in blood samples, and includes petro-chemicals and pesticides.

Diagnos-Techs, Inc.
6620 S. 192nd Place, Building J
Kent, WA 98032
800-878-3787

Lab does a wide range of tests on gastrointestinal function and saliva hormones.

Doctor's Data Laboratories, Inc.
3755 Illinois Avenue
St. Charles, IL 60174
800-323-2784

DDL specializes in mineral and heavy metal—mercury, lead, and so on—testing on blood, urine, and hair, and has also branched off into gastrointestinal testing.

Great Smokies/Genova Diagnostic Laboratory
63 Zillicoa Street
Asheville, NC 28801
800-522-4762

They are the original developer of GI testing with the CDSA (Comprehensive Digestive Stool Analysis) to assess function and the microbe environment (bacteria, yeast, and parasites). They also do mineral and metal testing, saliva hormone testing, and a detoxification profile.

Immunosciences Lab, Inc.
8693 Wilshire Boulevard, Suite #200
Beverly Hills, CA 90211
800-950-4686

This innovative lab does a wide variety of testing, including antibodies to viruses.

Meridian Valley Laboratory
801 SW 16th Street, Suite #126
Renton, WA 98055
425-271-8689

Meridian does a food allergy (antibody) test, saliva hormones, and many other health-related tests.

Metametrix Medical Laboratory
4855 Peachtree Industrial Boulevard,
Suite #201
Nocross, GA 30092
800-221-4640

This lab does a food allergy test and many others.

Parisitology Center, Inc. (PCI)
903 South Rural Road
#101-318 Tempe, AZ 85281
480-767-2522

PCI specializes in parasite evaluation on stool tests.

Doris Rapp, MD
www.DrRapp.com

Dr. Rapp is an environmental pediatric allegist focusing on the toxicity of our world. She has referral resources and good information on her site.

SUPPLEMENT COMPANIES WITH DETOXIFICATION PRODUCTS

Alacer Corporation
19631 Pauling
Foothill Ranch, CA 92610
800-854-0249

They make the well-known Emergen-C products, the powders with vitamin C, plus other vitamins and minerals in a variety of flavors.

Allergy Research Group/Nutricology
400 Preda Street
San Leandro, CA 94577
800-545-9960

ARG makes full-range, high-quality, hypoallergenic products and is known for its Vitamin C powder and Anti-Ox (antioxidant).

ApotheCure
13720 Midway Road, Suite 109
Dallas, TX 75244
800-969-6601

This is a compounding pharmacy used by physicians to order special products to support detoxification and other health issues.

Blessed Herbs
109 Bare Plains Road
Oakham, MA 01068
800-489-4372
www.blessedherbs.com

Douglas Laboratories
P.O. Box 8583
Pittsburgh, PA 15220
800-245-4440

They make a wide range of nutritional products, including many that support detoxification.

Klamath Blue-Green
P.O. Box 1626
Mt. Shasta, CA 96067
800-327-1956

This company is known for their algae products, which I commonly use in my Detox programs.

Metagenics
971 Calle Negocio
San Clemente, CA 92672
800-692-9400

This is a well-known company for practitioners, and they create a full line of high-quality, well-tested products for health and detoxification. Their line of Ultra-Clear products was created by Dr. Jeff Bland.

NeoGen Research Corporation
1005 Terminal Way, Suite 110
Reno, NV 89502
775-326-5741

They focus on a breakthrough antioxidant supplement, R-Lipoic Acid.

NF Formulas
805 SE Sherman
Portland, OR 97214
800-547-4871

This company makes a wide variety of products, including some for Detox.

Pure Body Institute
230 S. Olive Street
Ventura, CA 93001
800-952-7873

This company specializes in detox herbal formulas, one bottle for body and cell detox and the other for colon detox. I have used these successfully for many years.

Thorne Research
901 Triangle Drive
Sandpoint, ID 97030
800-869-9705

Thorne is well known for its line of products and its focus on detoxification.

Zand Herbal Formulas
1722 14th St, Suite 230
Boulder, CO 80302
800-800-0405

Zand makes good herbal products including its 7-day Detox formula.

PRACTITIONERS, FACILITIES, AND SPAS

Spa Bar
www.spa-bar.com
Owner: Galen Yuen
Spa Director: Taran Collis
246 Second Street
San Francisco, CA 94105
415-975-0888

The Spa Bar in downtown San Francisco is the first in a chain opening in airports and malls across the country in the next year. They offer detoxifying treatments such as lymphatic and Swedish massage, herbal and seaweed wraps, and salt scrubs. The virtue of the Spa Bar is that you do not need an appointment ahead of time. You may stop in and be treated on the spot. Daniella has been to the San Francisco location and was impressed with the quality of service. I believe these spas will become more popular as we prioritize a relaxed lifestyle to maintain our mental and physical health. Detox is really in!

Calistoga, California is a great place for Detox Therapies. Here are our two favorite Calistoga places:

Calistoga Spa
www.calistogaspa.com
1006 Washington
Calistoga, CA 94515
866-822-5772

I have been going to this wonderful healing and renovated resort for more than twenty-five years. I sometimes write and have meetings there, but mostly go to enjoy the wonderful pools, nice rooms with kitchenettes, and the quaint town of Calistoga. And their rates are quite reasonable as well as the costs for mud bathes and massage. Clean and well maintained.

Indian Springs
www.IndianSpringsCalistoga.com
1712 Lincoln Avenue
Calistoga, CA 94515
707-942-4913

Indian Springs spa has been operating since 1862, and Daniella says it's a real clean spa and her personal mecca, which she visits twice a year to relax, rejuvenate, and rebuild. They have an Olympic size swimming pool of pure mineral water and mud baths that pull toxins from the body. They also offer facials and massages and have cottages for guests to rent.

Other spas, health resorts, and healing waters for cities and areas around the country can be found on Spa Finders at ww.spafinder.com.

Spa Finder
www.spafinder.com
800-255-7727

Hot Springs
Hotsprings.org
800-SPA-CITY

Arkansas has many non-sulfur hot springs.

In Northern California, there are many other natural hot springs and spas. These include: Harbin Hot Springs, Orr Hot Springs, Wilbur Hot Springs, and Vichy Hot Springs in Ukiah. You can also find more exotic spas and springs in *Spa Magazine* and online. Sonoma Mission Inn is a full spa and resort that is quite elegant.

There are also other hot springs and resorts, such as We Care Spa in Desert Hot Springs, California and New Age Spa in Neversick, New York.

Tassajara Zen Mountain Center
www.sfzc.org
Tassajara Reservations
300 Page Street
San Francisco, CA 94102
831-659-2229
415-865-1899

Tassajara, Zen Mind Temple (Zenshin-ji), is a Zen Buddhist community established by San Francisco Zen Center in 1966. Their hot springs were used by the Esselen Indians, and it has been a hot springs resort from the 1860s. From May through August, Tassajara offers guest practice and work-study programs, workshops, and retreats as well as individual accommodations for vacationing guests. For the rest of the year, September through April, the monastery is closed to the public so that students of Zen Buddhism can engage in traditional monastic training periods. Reservations are absolutely required, even for day guests.

The Oaks at Ojai
www.oaksspa.com
572 N. Indian Canyon Drive
Ojai, CA 93023
800-753-OAKS (6257)

The Palms at Palm Springs
122 E. Ojai Avenue
Palm Springs, CA 92262
800-753-PALM (7256)
www.palmsspa.com

These are wonderful spa for weight loss and health improvement with their full exercise programs and their low-calorie, tasty food.

Canyon Ranch Health Resorts
Tucson, AZ and Lenox, MA in the Berkshires
800-742-9000

The Canyon ranch resorts are well known for their elegance, good food, and beautiful settings. I have lectured at both of them.

Tree of Life Rejuvenation Center
www.treeoflife.nu
Gabriel Cousens, M.D.
P.O. Box 1080
Patagonia, AZ 85624
520-394-2520

Dr. Cousens is a masterful doctor who runs his practice and retreat center and also offers fasting programs throughout the year.

Ten Thousand Waves
www.tenthousandwaves.com
3451 Hyde Park Road
Santa Fe, NM 87501
505-992-5025 for informaton
505-982-9304 for reservations

This well-reputed spa offers steams, saunas, massages, and relaxation at its beautifully appointed Japanese style complex. Lodging includes individual cabins. See the spa's comprehensive website for more details.

Bauman College
www.baumancollege.org
P.O. Box 940
Penngrove, CA 94951
800-987-7530

Dr. Ed Bauman is a long-time friend and runs this nutritional certification school in Northern California. He also runs some fasting retreats and is quite knowledgeable in this process.

Khalsa Medical Clinic
www.khalsamedical.com
435 North Bedford Drive
Beverly Hills, CA 90210
310-274-6200

This is a practice by Soran Singh Khalsa, M.D., an integrated internal medicine doctor.

Optimum Health Institute of San Diego
www.optimalhealth.org
6970 Central Avenue
Lemon Grove, CA 91945
800-993-4325 or 619-464-3346

They also have a location in Austin, TX. OHI specializes in "live foods" like raw and sprouted beans, nuts and seeds, as well as intestinal detoxification. The program emphasizes self-discipline and the value of taking responsibility for oneself.

Sanoviv
Rosararita Beach
Baja, Mexico
800-SANOVIV

A lovely modern, electromagnetic hotel right over the beach with ocean sounds off every room. A full spa, swimming, and progressive medical clinic for alternative, biologic medicine, some not offered in the United States. Like the Optimum Health Institutes, they serve wholesome, mostly raw foods, and sprouts as they encourage live, vital foods.

National Acupuncture Detoxification Association (NADA)
P.O. Box 1927
Vancouver, WA 98668
888-765-NADA
email: nadaclear@aol.com

NADA is an organization of licensed acupuncturists who are trained in detoxification

National Health Association
www.anhs.org
813-855-6607

Formerly referred to as the American Natural Hygiene Society, they have a list of practitioners who are trained in natural hygiene diets and water fasting.

Susan Smith Jones
www.susansmithjones.com
Health Unlimited and Celebrate Life!
P.O. Box 49396
Los Angeles, CA 90049

Susan is a friend, an author and teacher, but not a practitioner. She teaches at UCLA, and her books are very inspirational for fasting and healthy living.

Azure Acres
2264 Green Hill Rd.
Sebastopol, CA 95472
800-222-7292 or 707-823-3385

This center offers a 28-day residential treatment program for chemical dependency.

St. Helena Health Center at St. Helena Hospital
www.sthelenahospital.org
Deer Park, CA 94576
800-454-HOPE (4673)

This center offers alcohol and drug recovery programs in a nice setting away from the big cities.

Sierra Tucson
39580 S. Lago del Oro Parkway
Tucson, AZ 85739
800-842-4487

This 30-day, in-patient, dual-diagnosis facility treats substance abuse, mental health issues, eating disorders, gambling, trauma, and sexual compulsivity.

True North Health Center
www.healthpromoting.com
Alan Goldhamer, D.C., Director
4310 Lichau Road
Penngrove, CA 94951
707-792-2325
707-586-5544 (fax)

This center is based on natural hygiene approach and oversees water fasting programs in treatment of medical issues.

HOTLINES

Center for National Help Hotline
800-662-4357 (HELP) • www.drughelp.org
Main number for all kinds of substance abuse problems.

Children of Alcoholics Foundation
800-943-7646 • www.coaf.org

Service of National Help Line
800-662-HELP

National Clearinghouse for Alcohol and Drug Information
800-729-6686 • www.health.org
Information resource and referral service.

National Council on Alcoholism and Drug Dependence
800-622-2255 • www.neadd.org
This help line offers counseling and treatment options for teens and parents.

National Acupuncture Detox Association (NADA)
888-765-6232 • www.acudetox.com

MAIL ORDER COMPANIES AND OTHER RESOURCES

Natural and Organic Foods

Many websites offer the same foods found at co-ops and whole foods markets. These are just a few: www.truefoodsonline.com and www.nspiredfoods.com

Diamond Organics
www.diamondorganics.com
888-674-2642 or 888-ORGANIC

This company has a wide range of organic produce and products available through its website and catalog.

Guilt-Free Cookie Book
P.O. Box 1274
Ketchum, ID 83340

Written by Daniella Chace and Connie Aronson, a highly respected personal fitness trainer and "cookie guru" from Sun Valley, Idaho, this compilation of their favorite "healthy cookie" recipes incorporates nutritious alternative sweeteners such as barley malt syrup, brown rice syrup, stevia, turbinado sugar, date sugar, and fruit sweeteners. Each chapter contains nutrition information, recipes, and tips for baking delicious healthy cookies to fulfill your own cravings and for entertaining. To order a copy, send $14 to Connie Aronson at the above P.O. Box.

Golden Moon Tea, Ltd.
Golden Moon Tea is owned by an old friend of Daniella's, Cindy Knotts, who imports Black, Green, Oolong, and White Teas from around the globe. They specialize in hand plucked whole-leaf tea from the world's finest gardens. High in antioxidants and rich in antibacterial cancer-prevention properties, tea is a healthier alternative to coffee as a daily ritual. Online orders through www.goldenmoontea.com

Garden of Life
www.gardenlifeusa.com
562-748-2477

This company makes Perfect food, which is a green powder consisting of dried green vegetables, phytoplanktons such as Spirulina, chlorella and dulse, vitamin C, and probiotics. They also make a probiotic powder called Primal Defense that has a wide range of microflora. The products are available through markets, co-ops and health food stores as well as on their website.

Green Vibrant
www.vibranthealth.org
800-242-1835

This green powder supplement contains alfalfa, chlorella, pectin, and blue green algae among other nutritious ingredients.

Maranatha
www.maranathanutbutters.com
This natural food products company makes excellent organic nut butters.

Kettle
www.kettlefoods.com
This company makes high-quality organic nut butters. Many of their products are wheat-free and guaranteed gluten-free. They test for aflatoxins in their peanut butter and most of their products are GMO-free, meaning they are not genetically engineered.

Ancient Sun Nutrition Inc.
www.ancientsuninc.com
President: Clive Adams
Algae expert: Michelle Davis
P.O. Box 7555
Asheville, NC 28802
800-877-428-0509
828-651-9290

This algae company has crystal manna algae products, 100 percent organic, wild crafted, fresh dried blue green algae from Klamath Lake. Their algae is available as capsules or tablets in bottles and as flakes in bulk. They also have the mood enhancing, inflammation reducing blue manna, which is composed of the concentrated blue pigment from the algae.

J.P. Durga
www.jpdurga.com
P.O. Box 65346
Port Ludlow, WA 98365-0346
360-437-0826

This small natural body care products company makes the most effective all-natural deodorant that we have found to date. They also make exceptionally high-quality lip balm, all-body moisturizer, massage cream, shampoo, and soap.

Laural Naturals
lauralnaturals@excite.com
543 North Barr Road
Port Angeles, WA 98362
360-452-9197

Laural's products are made from goat milk and essential oils, beeswax, honey, and royal jelly. They carry a full line of soaps, oil bars, bath salts, cold cream, foot balm, and salves. They even carry a natural buy repellent.

www.elementemporium.com
For education clothing and other products co-designed by Dr. Haas. These include Sole Sox, the Acu-T, the Chakra-T, and others. Run by Bethany ArgISLE of ArgISLE Enterprises, this website ships all of Dr. Haas's books.

OTHER BOOKS BY DR. ELSON HAAS

Staying Healthy with Nutrition: The Complete Guide to Diet and Nutritional Medicine

The definitive resource for understanding the significant role of nutrition in our health. It is used as a home and school textbook and reference guide. Look for the fully updated and resourced edition in autumn of 2004. 1,200 pages.

Staying Healthy with the Seasons (Newly Updated 21st Century Edition)

Dr. Haas's popular first book, revised for its twenty-seventh printing, is a classic, integrating Eastern and Western health systems with practical guidelines for nutrition, herbology, and exercise. 252 pages.

A Cookbook for All Seasons (this book may be transformed into *The After Detox Diet Plan: Healthy Eating for Life*)

Dr. Haas gives us expert guidelines for a healthy, transition from his Detox diet and a clear plan for changing our focus to fresh, home-cooked meals, attuned to the seasons, with menu plans and over 150 recipes. 224 pages.

The Staying Healthy Shopper's Guide: Feed Your Family Safely

An important book that helps us understand the chemicals in our food and life, and how they affect our health. Clear guidelines in what to avoid and what to shop for, including the healthy feeding of our young ones. 224 pages.

These above books are available from your local bookstore, or direct from Celestial Arts, P.O. Box 7123, Berkeley, CA 94707. For VISA, MasterCard, and American Express orders call 800-841-BOOK.

Other books by Dr. Haas include:

Vitamins for Dummies (with Christopher Hobbs, LAc) IDG Books Worldwide, Foster City, Ca, 1999.

The False Fat Diet (with Cameron Struth) Ballantine Books, New York, 2001.

Edu-Products (co-designed with Dr. Haas) These t-shirts and reflexology socks are available through www.elementemporium.com and on the telephone at 415-455-4656.

You may contact Dr. Elson Haas:
www.elsonhaas.com
Preventive Medical Center of Marin, Inc.
25 Mitchell Boulevard., Suite 8
San Rafael, CA 94903
415-472-2343
415-472-7636 (fax)
email: emhaas@sonic.net

OTHER BOOKS BY DANIELLA CHACE

Bread Machine Baking for Better Health: Prima Publishing, 1994. (Coauthored with Maureen Keane.)

This book is especially helpful for those who want to bake breads for special dietary needs as you will find recipes for wheat-free, gluten-free, or dairy-free breads.

Grains for Better Health: Prima Publishing, 1994. (Coauthored with Maureen Keane.)

This ancient grain cookbook offers delicious recipes for cooking with wholesome grains such as teff, quinoa, amaranth, spelt, and kamut.

What To Eat if You Have Cancer: Contemporary Books, 1996.
The What To Eat if You Have Cancer Cookbook: Contemporary Books, 1996. (Coauthored with Maureen Keane.)

These best-selling books address nutrition for the prevention and treatment of cancer. The text defines cancer and its biological process and makes specific scientifically based nutritional recommendations, while the cookbook offers simple and delicious recipes based on these studies.

Smoothies for Life: Prima Publishing, 1998. (Coauthored with Amy Boyer.)

This popular recipe book guides the reader through an array of smoothie ingredients, their nutritional value and health benefits, and how to combine ingredients to make delicious and nutrient-dense drinks.

What To Eat if You Have Heart Disease: Contemporary Books, 1998.
What To Eat if You Have Heart Disease Cookbook: NTC/Contemporary Publishing Group, 2000. (Coauthored with Maureen Keane.)

These books offer a plan for choosing the best foods to help combat heart disease as well as information on how and why nutritional therapy helps heart disease patients. The book also includes a clear and concise overview of the disease, specific dietary plans, and information on nutritional supplements.

What To Eat if You Have Diabetes: Contemporary Books, 1999.
What To Eat if You Have Diabetes Cookbook: NTC/Contemporary/Ingram, 1999. (Coauthored with Maureen Keane.)

This easy-to-follow program helps those with hypoglycemia or diabetes control blood sugar levels, while this cookbook offers delectable recipes based on the program.

The RV Cookbook: Prima Publishing, 2002. (Coauthored with Amy Boyer.)

If you are one of the record numbers of Americans hitting the open road in a recreational vehicle, these healthy and mouthwatering recipes will help you stay healthy on the road.

You may contact Daniella Chace for private individual nutrition consultation or speaking engagements through her website: DaniellaChace, M.S., C.N., Nutritionist www.daniellachace.com

Glossary

◆

Agar-Agar

Agar-Agar, pronounced AH-gahr-AH-gahr is a product made from seaweed that is dried and powdered and sold as a thickening or gelling agent. It is tasteless and comes in the form of blocks, powder, and strands. It is widely available in Asian markets, health food stores, and through mail order sources. It is a vegan alternative to gels made from animal by-products and a good dietary source of calcium and iron.

Balsamic Vinegar

This Italian vinegar, pronounced bal-SAH-mihk VIHN-ih-ger, is made from white Trebbiano grape juice that gets its dark color and pungent flavor from the barrels it is aged in. For those who are sensitive to sulfites, be aware that many balsamic vinegars contains sulfites to inhibit the growth of flavor detracting bacteria.

Basmati Rice

Pronounced bahs-MAH-tee, it is a long grained rice with a fine texture that has a nutlike flavor and aroma.

Cold Pressed

The term cold pressed refers to the process used to extract culinary oils such as olive oil. Cold pressed is healthier than the common chemical extraction process. Heat makes oils become rancid so the fat soluble vitamins are lost in the extraction process if the machines heat up. When the term *cold pressed* is used on an oil label it means care was taken to keep the process cold to preserve the natural nutrients in the oil.

Dulse

Dulse (duhlss) is coarse-textured, red seaweed with a pungent, briny flavor. It grows around the British Isles and has a rubbery texture even when dried. Some Irish use it like a chewing tobacco. It is primarily used as flavoring in soups and as a condiment on salads and grains. It is available dried, granulated, powdered, or in sheets. It is nutritionally rich in minerals, magnesium, fiber, rich in vitamin C and beta-carotene, potassium, calcium, iron, and iodine. It is also high in trace minerals and used as a treatment for thyroid disorders.

Flaxseed
Raw flaxseed powder, flaxseed oil, and whole flax seeds are all widely available. Flax is added to smoothies to add soluble and insoluble fiber and essential fatty acids. When you buy flaxseed products they should have a fresh nutty flavor. If the product starts to smell rancid or fishy, throw it out. Refrigerate the oil and keep the whole flaxseed and ground flaxseed in the freezer and it will stay fresh longer. If you have whole flaxseeds, they should be ground before you add them to a smoothie. Use a food processor, blender, or a coffee grinder for the job.

Ghee
Ghee is clarified butter. It can be purchased at natural grocery stores or made at home. To make ghee, simply melt butter and skim off all the impurities that float to the top of the oil. The transparent golden liquid that is left in the pan is "purified butter" or ghee.

Ginger
Gingerroot is sold fresh in the produce department of most markets. It is a digestive aid useful in treating nausea, morning sickness, and motion sickness. Gingerroot has been used as a digestive and circulatory stimulant for thousands of years.

Glutathione
This amino acid is an important source of sulfur for the body. Sulfur-containing compounds function as detoxifying agents by combining with toxic substances, making them water soluble so that they can be excreted thought the kidneys. Glutathione is a sulfur-containing compound that is found in watermelon, strawberries, avocados, and carrots.

Green Tea
Caffeine-free green tea, green tea extract, and leaf tea are all available. Green tea is rich in antioxidants and cancer-fighting, naturally occurring plant chemicals.

Hijiki
Pronounced hee-JEE-kee, it is a sea vegetable. It is a flavorful addition to soups and stews, dressings, and dips. Hijiki has a high mineral content, ten times more calcium by volume than milk, cheese, or other dairy products. It is also high in iron, protein, beta-carotene, B_1, and B_{12}. Available dried, this black seaweed has a slight anise character and nutty aroma. Usually dried into skinny strips, it is available in both dried and fresh varieties at Asian markets, health food stores, and mail order companies.

Jicama

Pronounced HEE-ka-mah, it is a mild, very low calorie, watery, root vegetable that can be added to either vegetable or fruit combinations.

Kelp

Nutrients—Kelp contains sodium, potassium, calcium, iodine, and other trace minerals and vitamins.

Health Benefits—Easily assimilated form of minerals. This is particularly beneficial for those with mineral deficiencies that have developed from a long-term fast food diet. It can be purchased dried, granulated, or powdered and added in small quantities to smoothies.

Kombu

Kombu, pronounced kohm-boo, is a sea vegetable that grows in long, dark brown fronds up to 15 feet in length. It is harvested and sun-dried and folded into sheets. It is used to make a flavorful broth, as flavoring in soups, bean dishes, and longer-cooking stews. It can be purchased dried in packages and stored indefinitely unopened. After opening, store in a cool dry place for up to six months. Kombu is a rich source of beta-carotene, B_2, C, calcium, and iodine.

Kudzu

This tuberous root, pronounced KOOD-zoo, is pulverized and dried to produce kudzu powder, which is used for thickening soups and sauces and stews. It is high in fiber, protein, vitamins A and D, and widely available in Asian markets and health food stores.

Maple Syrup

Real pure maple syrup is from the sap of maple trees and is rich in potassium and calcium. Pure maple syrup has a dark brown color and rich maple flavor. There are unhealthy imitation syrups made with just a small amount of real maple and corn syrup, which do not taste nearly as good. Be aware that the sugar-free maple syrups are usually made from chemicals such as aspartame, which are unhealthy and taste like synthetic chemicals. The highest quality products are organic and 100 percent pure maple syrup. The organic label in this case assures you that the producers have not used formaldehyde pellets or other additives in the processing.

Microflora

Gastrointestinal (GI) flora such as acidophilus and other positive digestive bacteria are also known as probiotics, beneficial microflora, and intestinal flora. Dysbiosis is the term used to describe an imbalance in microbial populations. Reinoculation or reflorastation is the replacement of microflora with supplements.

Millet

Millet has a light and delicate flavor similar to toasted cashew nuts. It is a good source of protein as well as B-vitamins and the minerals magnesium, zinc, copper, and iron. Millet is sold in boxes and in bins for bulk buying. It has a long shelf life, but like all grains, it should be kept in a sealed container and stored in a dark cool place. Raw millet can be stored for up to 6 months. Cooked millet can be stored for up to three days in the refrigerator. Millet is an extremely versatile grain. It can be steamed directly or toasted in a dry skillet before steaming. Cooked millet makes an excellent porridge or pudding. It can also be served as a pilaf, stuffing, or as an addition to soups and green salads. Raw, it can be added to other grains as a crunchy topping.

Muesli

This healthy mix of dried fruits and raw or toasted grains was developed by a Swiss nutritionist near the end of the 19th century. It has since become a popular breakfast cereal in Europe and the United States. Many people enjoy Muesli soaked in apple juice for several hours before eating to soften the grains for easier digestion.

Natural Tobacco

There are a few companies making what is considered "natural" tobacco, meaning that it is either organic or grown without synthetic agricultural chemicals. Also, natural tobacco should not have any chemicals added to the tobacco after harvest. Most tobacco products are not grown organically and contain not only agricultural chemicals but also up to 400 other additives. Also be aware that most cigarette papers are treated with dangerous chemicals to slow down the burning of the paper. There are clean papers that are not treated and therefore a much healthier alternative, which are available through companies such as Rizla.com

Nori

Nori, pronounced NOH-ree, is generally used for wrapping sushi and making rice balls in Japan. It is 48 percent protein by dry-weight and a rich source of beta-carotene, thiamine, niacin, calcium, iron, and trace minerals. It is the most easily digestible of the seaweeds. Paper-thin sheets are made from the seaweed, which can range in color from dark green to dark purple to black and have a sweet subtle ocean flavor. The sheets can be toasted over a flame or purchased pre-toasted (labeled yakinori). Nori sheets are generally used as a sushi wrap and as flavoring for soups and grains.

Organic

As of October 2002, the National Organic Standards Board has clearly defined the term *organic*. For any product or produce to be labeled organic it must be grown without chemical herbicides, pesticides, fertilizers, and without genetic engineering (genetic alteration or gene splicing).

OTC

OTC is the abbreviation for Over the Counter drugs and other medications sold directly to the consumer rather than through a pharmacist with a doctor's prescription.

Pears

Pears are very nutritious containing potassium, pectins, hemicellulose, vitamin C, folic acid, potassium, manganese, and selenium. Pears contain plant estrogens, along with the antioxidant and anti-carcinogen glutathione, which is recommended for the prevention of high blood pressure and stroke. Hemicellulose is an indigestible complex carbohydrate or fiber source that promotes the beneficial intestinal flora necessary for digestion and proper elimination.

Pectin

Pectin is a soluble fiber that is beneficial in regulating blood sugar, removing metals and toxins in the digestive tract, and reducing elevated cholesterol levels. Packaged pectin is generally extracted from citrus or apples, but is also found in carrots, beets, bananas, and citrus fruits.

Probiotics

See Microflora.

Quinoa

Quinoa, pronounced keen-wa, is a protein and nutrient-rich grain. Quinoa has a mild flavor and can be substituted for recipes calling for couscous, bulgur, buckwheat, or millet. It can be used in soups, puddings, and as a topping for salads or as hot breakfast porridge. Quinoa contains more oils than most grains so it has a limited shelf life. In warm weather, store quinoa in a sealed container in the refrigerator to prevent rancidity.

Sea Salt

When purchasing sea salt look for high-quality sea salts with iodine added. For many people iodized salt is their main source of iodine, which is essential for proper thyroid function. Sea salt contains minerals that table salt is lacking. Table salt also may contain the chemicals used to remove the minerals such as sulfuric acid and chlorine as well as anti-caking agents such as ferrocynide, yellow prussiate of soda, and tri-calcium phosphate.

Spirulina

Algae has been shown to protect the immune system and lower serum cholesterol levels, and contains easily assimilated minerals. This algae is an excellent source of many B vitamins, iron, and trace minerals.

Stevia

An acceptable sweetener throughout the detox diet, this sweetener is made from the leaves of a plant from South America. It does not appear to raise blood sugar levels or increase fungal growth such as Candida.

Tahini

Tahini is the paste of ground sesame seeds with a creamy texture and fresh nutty flavor. It is used in many Middle Eastern dishes such as hummus and can be added to salad dressings, smoothies, dips, and sauces. It is high in protein and contains fat-soluble vitamins, calcium, protein, and fiber. There are several types of tahini on the grocery store shelves to choose from. Toasted sesame seed tahini is preferred as it has a deeper smoky flavor.

Wakame

Wakame, pronounced wah-KAH-meh, is an olive-colored algae that grows in wing-like fronds up to twenty inches long in shallow water and up to twenty feet long in deeper waters. The dark brown variety is more strongly flavored. Wakame is high in calcium, iron, beta-carotene, niacin, and protein. It is available through Asian markets, health food stores, and through mail order companies.

Whole Foods

Foods in their whole form that are as unrefined as possible are considered "whole foods": whole wheat bread versus refined white bread, steel-cut oats versus quick-cooking, rolled, pre-cooked oats, dates versus date sugar, for example. Of course, this is also the name of a popular chain of food stores.

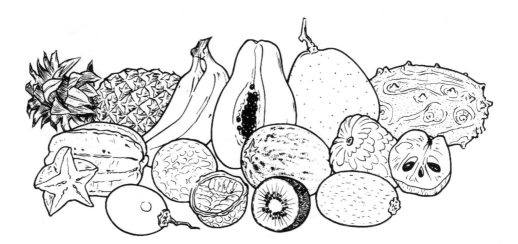

Index

◆